FOOTBALL WIFE

Coming of Age with the NFL as Mrs. Karl Kassulke

Jan Thatcher Adams, MD

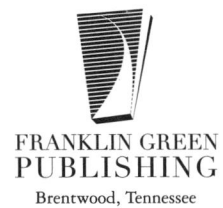

FRANKLIN GREEN
PUBLISHING
Brentwood, Tennessee

FOOTBALL WIFE
PUBLISHED BY FRANKLIN GREEN PUBLISHING
500 Wilson Pike Circle, Suite 100
Brentwood, Tennessee 37027
www.franklingreenpublishing.com

ISBN 978-1-936487-04-2

Printed in the United States of America

1 2 3 4 5 6 7 8 9 10—15 14 13 12 11

Cover design by Clifford Koidahl, Minneapolis, Minnesota
Cover photography by Judy Olausen, Minneapolis, Minnesota

To my wonderful sons
KURT and KORY
who lived these days and years with me
and brought sunshine to my life

In Memoriam

Karl Kassulke

Otto Kassulke

Leona Kassulke

Kathy Kassulke

Rev. Willard Kassulke

Mildred Thatcher

Howard Thatcher

Wally Hilgenberg

Earsall Macbee

Dr. Pearl Rosenberg

Dr. William Stromme

Rose Embry

Dr. Hilmer Carlson

Dr. Albert Sullivan

Contents

Acknowledgments

$\mathcal{L}$IKE EVERY author, I cannot begin to thank the many wonderful people who have played so many critical roles in my life and writing, both now and in the period this book covers. To all of you, I am forever grateful.

First, I must acknowledge Dmitri Gerasimenko, my incredible husband and my true better half, without whom I would not even be alive. My deep thanks to Jim Klobuchar for his sage advice that led me to Ian Graham Leask, my superb writing coach. I am deeply grateful to Ron Pitkin for walking me through the publishing of my first book.

The University of Minnesota Medical School shaped my life and career, and I am so thankful they gave me a chance to be a doctor at a time when women doctors, especially married women with children, were a rarity. At the university, I remain ever grateful to Dr. Pearl Rosenberg, Dr. Erskine Caperton, and Dr. Albert Sullivan.

My freshman year at Drake University on scholarship played a huge role in my life, and I am equally grateful to my parents, Karl Kassulke's family, Bud Grant, the Minnesota Vikings and the Vikings wives, Boone, Iowa, and all of Minnesota.

I want to acknowledge the ongoing encouragement I have received from my writer friends: Sarah Susanka, Antonia Felix, and Gloria Karpinski. And in the publication and publicity of the book, I would be lost without the input of Lee Gessner, Pat Lindquist, and Ed Curtis.

Finally, my beloved sons, Kurt and Kory Kassulke, are part of the reason I wrote this chronicle. They are the best and most special blessing that emerged from the challenge and delight of those years.

Foreword

*A*s a teenager, I had an unusual and abrupt introduction into adulthood and marriage. Besides all the usual responsibilities of marriage and family, I was in a celebrity marriage to Karl Kassulke, a Minnesota Vikings football player, and neither my husband nor I had any idea what that would really mean to us. When my marriage failed and ended in divorce after nine years, I buried all my emotions away and never really dealt with them.

My life went on, and I grew to understand that all the difficulties that arise in a person's life are the stuff of growth and maturity, so Karl Kassulke remained in my heart for the many good things he was. And I remained grateful for the time we shared together and for our two beautiful sons.

Then, in 2008, thirty-five years after the divorce, two traumatic events stirred up all the old emotions. I nearly died from cancer, and Karl did die from a sudden heart attack. His funeral brought everything to the fore again, and it was clear that now was the time for me to actually achieve closure on these long-ago events.

Since I was a writer by avocation, I started to write the story of this fabled and failed marriage, intending it to be a journal of sorts. The more I wrote, however, the more I understood that the problems central to the failure of my marriage are still very much issues today. Drug abuse, alcoholism, codependency, adult children of alcoholics, infidelity, the cult of celebrity, and the recent devastating research chronicling the results of recurrent concussions among NFL players are all very important societal topics and can always use more light on them.

And so I decided to write and publish *Football Wife*. It's not just another kiss-and-tell book. There are real issues here, timeless issues that played out for me in a very public arena. Writing the book was therapeutic; Karl's memory is in a peaceful place for me now. Since both Karl and I dedicated ourselves in later years to the service of others, it is my hope that *Football Wife* can be an inspirational read as well.

NOTE: Please see the glossary on page 270 for definitions and clarifications of terms as they are used in this book.

Prologue

~~~~~~

*B*ESIDES RECEIVING TWO BEAUTIFUL sons from my marriage to football hero Karl Kassulke, I also acquired a ripping case of the clap. That was a sickening life lesson, harder than I could have imagined. Thirty-five years have passed since then, and most of my memories of that marriage have, like many of life's troubles, faded to the fun, passion, and unique experiences we shared—but a few still remain traumatic. The majority of the difficulties have become mild background chatter, but I will never be without reminders of a few whoppers. However, as one ages, parents, lovers, siblings, and friends die and stir up surprising reflections. In our coming of age together, Karl and I experienced a juicy and painful marriage that could not last, although love was there—a long-ago chapter in my life.

October 28, 2008: Karl is dead, stricken with a sudden, midsentence, and totally unexpected heart attack at the age of sixty-seven. He'd recently been given an all clear after a cardiac exam. Our sons, forty-three-year-old Kurt and forty-one-year-old Kory, flew in from Los Angeles, California, and Wilmington, North Carolina, their respective homes. We drove together to the funeral home in Eagan, Minnesota, for Karl's visitation. I was surprised as we turned in to the parking lot to find relatively few parked cars there. Given Karl's forty-five years of Minnesota celebrity, I had expected to see hundreds of fans at his visitation, with a line out the door waiting to view his casket.

Instead, we entered the foyer and found no line at all. We weren't late. We arrived just after 6:00 p.m., with two hours to spare. Despite ten years of playing for the Minnesota Vikings, All-Pro status, and frequent ongoing attention after football due to his injury, his altruistic efforts in the community, and his story of Christian redemption, told in his autobiographical book, *Kassulke,* there was no line of patiently waiting, saddened people. I'd been to so many visitations with long lines, and I just didn't understand this. But I'd long since learned that life itself, and my ex-husband Karl, often present questions to which I have no answer.

Once in the viewing room, Kory, Kurt, and I moved forward past several clutches of folks chatting. Without identifying any of the people present or looking to either side, we approached the casket. I took a quick look at his carefully composed body, which didn't look much like Karl, and moved on.

Even though we'd been divorced for thirty-five years and hadn't seen each other very often during those years, Karl remained in my heart for his good traits and as the father of our sons. And though my years as a physician had resulted in seeing many people in death and had taught me to keep my emotions to myself, I was rocked to the core at this finality. Karl dead—my childhood sweetheart, always bursting with life and laughter—dead? It still feels impossible, even as I write.

And then again, the scientist, the rationalist in me never imagined that Karl would survive this long. It's an irony that after several years without communicating, I had shared a pleasant lunch with Karl and Sue, his wife, just a few weeks earlier, and Karl seemed fine—even in radiant spirits

Kurt and Kory, too, had no wish to linger at the casket. They moved over to be with twenty-nine-year-old Christopher, their half brother and Karl and Sue's son. They hadn't seen each other for years, and so they began to catch up. Then they moved about the room. Everyone recognized them and was happy to see them.

I chatted for a bit with Karl's widow, Sue, a nurse and a veteran of thirty-three years of marriage to him. Were it not for her loving care and attention all these years after the motorcycle accident, Karl, paralyzed with significant brain damage and in a wheelchair, would have had a much different life, not to mention a shorter one.

Then I moved to a foyer off the main room, where there were couches I could sit on. I'd just managed to get out of bed after nine months of suffering with a terrible cancer, radiation therapy to my head and neck, and nine hospitalizations from the side effects. I'd lost a hundred pounds, and I saw the shock on many faces at my appearance. I looked like I could easily be the next person in a casket! My blood pressure was dangerously low, and I was suffering from severe anemia due to the radiation therapy, so standing for any length of time was impossible.

As I rested and caught my breath, old friends from those long-gone days drifted over to talk. Many sat with me for long talks, and I was never alone. Several started in with medical conversations in the old comfortable way we had so many years earlier. Mary Hilgenberg told me that her husband Wally, a sixteen-year veteran of pro football at both linebacker and guard, had died the previous month. He had struggled for several years with a fatal degenerative brain disease, amyotrophic lateral sclerosis (ALS—Lou Gehrig's disease). Mary is a nurse, and I had been a physician for thirty-five years, so we had a technical talk about Wally's long decline with this terrible neurological disaster.

I had already looked around the visitation and had noticed that many of the former Vikings present seemed to be suffering from degenerative brain diseases, and I commented on this to Mary. She told me that Wally's brain had been sent to Boston University, where an extensive study is going on regarding the severe damage sustained from repeated concussions in football players. The study is clearly indicating these concussions cause a wide spectrum of long-term neurological problems for football players as they age, including fatal brain degeneration such as Wally's. She told me his brain had so many damaged areas, the researchers at Boston University were amazed he had stayed alive and functioning for as long as he did. I didn't comment on this much. I hadn't seen the study, so I wasn't sure if it factored in other contact sports, drug use, or other issues. I know Wally wasn't one of the Vikings I associated with drug or heavy alcohol use.

It was lovely to see Sue and John Campbell again. They were good friends, and John had had some health problems, though his brain seemed to be fine, and he looked fit. Sue had brought their children to me as their physician for a time many years ago, but I hadn't seen any of them for at least twenty-five years.

Throughout the evening, former players, friends, coaches, and staff moved over to where I sat and did what most folks do at funerals and visitations. They regaled me with funny stories about Karl, most of which occurred during our marriage. I enjoyed them but realized, truly for the first time, that there was a very large part of Karl's life I knew nothing about. Most of these stories were news to me, and I began to understand the huge extent of my own denial regarding our many years together.

Because of this, in the car on the way home I decided to read "the book." I call it "the book" because its presence in my life had been a constant reminder of those long-ago years. There has never been even a week since its publication in 1981 without someone mentioning it to me or my seeing it on a bookshelf somewhere.

Kassulke: The True Story of Minnesota Vikings' Star Karl Kassulke and the Accident That Changed His Life—For Good, by Karl Kassulke and Ron Pitkin, had been on my shelf since publication. The focus of the book is on Karl's redemption and evangelical Christian conversion later in life.

I hadn't read it. I hadn't even wanted to read it until now. I just hadn't wanted to revisit any of the pain or lost hopes of those years. I had neatly put them in a box and locked the lid. And knowing the book was written when Karl was severely brain damaged, I figured any items about our marriage, gleaned from sources who could not have known the inside workings of our life together (since I was not consulted), would not be accurate. And in order to shine the best possible light on Karl, I assumed that I would be somewhat demonized. Both assumptions proved accurate.

But Karl's death and visitation caused me to realize I hadn't achieved proper closure with that very important chapter of my life, and I'd finally have to finish it. Part of that closure would be reading Karl's book.

So the night before Karl's funeral, I took the book from the shelf and read it through in one sitting. What I learned was that I really didn't know much about Karl's life, even though we lived together and loved each other. He kept his wild life completely away from my knowledge, as much as possible, and I found I didn't know more than two of the colorful and crazy stories in the book.

It looks like he sure had fun with his hijinks, and apparently he also was fined a lot by Coach Bud Grant, who rightfully didn't appreciate all of Karl's prankster stuff (although he was very respectful of Karl's playing). I hoped all these entertaining stories were true, because Karl's life took a somber turn when he was first divorced and then paralyzed. A lot of the fun stopped very abruptly for him then.

But the issues and the pressures on celebrities and their families were touched upon gingerly in the book. The alcohol and drug use and their results (and the womanizing) are timeless problems and much in the media of late, and *Kassulke,* as many books about celebrities do, plays down the negatives, sometimes to a very big degree. But human nature does not change, although we know much more now about the results of chemical and alcohol addictions. And we can predict what happens to the psyche of a child or an adult who is a user or who loves a user. There are words to describe these outcomes and treatments to intervene and heal. None of this was much in evidence in the sixties and early seventies.

Nor were there many public consequences to these problems. Certainly the private lives of celebrities, sports figures, and politicians suffered, but these folks were generally protected by the media, the teams, and law enforcement from consequences that could have started them on the road to healing. For instance, were Karl living his life today as a pro football hero, he would be called out as a Tiger Woods by a relentless media and punished for his reckless driving and alcohol and drug use by at least DUIs and fines, if not worse.

Reading the book proved to be the final push I needed to write my own memoir—a memoir that is not intended to be a biography of Karl

Kassulke, but rather an account of my own life lessons and stories. So Karl will populate this memoir writ large as my husband during the huge shifts in American culture and in our relationship with each other.

The culture was remarkable because ideas and mores shifted from conservative to ultraliberal, at least among the young, within a few years. Clothing went from modest to outrageous, and experimentation with alternative sexual ideas and drugs quickly became the norm, rather than the exception. Music took a quantum leap from big bands and Johnny Mathis to the Beatles and then acid rock. Women threw away their girdles, then their bras.

And together Karl and I grew in stature within our areas of expertise. Karl played remarkable, entertaining football and was rewarded with awards and respect for his pains. At the same time, I was educating myself to be one of the few female doctors practicing medicine at the time and was raising our sons. Though there seems to have been some talk about us being in competition during our marriage, I was never aware of that. I only knew that, despite the major issues that tore us apart, we never stopped being supportive and proud of each other.

For me, funerals are always a time for reflection and grief. Besides stimulating my decision to restart my stalled writing, Karl's funeral caused me to realize how much more there was yet to discover about having come of age while living with a man who loved me but did not share his life with me.

Also poignant was the fact that after Kurt and Kory moved away from Minneapolis, they didn't see their dad that often. They lived on the coasts, and Karl didn't travel, due to his condition. So for twenty years or more, their times with their dad were rare and brief. Mostly they had kept in contact by telephone.

However, Kurt and his wife, Shelley, and their two daughters, five-year-old Akira and one-year-old Asha (whom Karl had never seen), had traveled to Minnesota in September 2008.

They came specifically because it looked like I might die.

Karl's wife, Sue, took advantage of Kurt's family's visit to invite us all, including Dmitri, my third husband, to have lunch together at one of her favorite restaurants, and we all went. It was a fine time, though it was difficult for me to sit for very long. Karl glowed with the pleasure of meeting his grandchildren and seeing his beloved son again. Within a month, Karl was dead.

So, after the visitation, I took a short sleep and began a long read to educate myself about the fullness of the man I had loved and married so many years ago. Thus wiser, I drove with Dmitri and my sons to Karl's church in Eagan for his funeral. There was a larger crowd at the funeral, though still the church wasn't packed. Kurt and Kory moved to the front of the church to sit with Karl's family, and Dmitri and I sat farther back. I didn't make any move toward Karl's casket, though it was still open. I'd seen enough of him in death—I needed to keep my last memories of him more vital.

At the funeral I saw many more Vikings players and their wives. I didn't recognize them all, but they recognized me. Two old friends broke out crying at the sight of me and hugged me tight, hoping I wouldn't die too.

The church service was sweet, with background music playing much of the time on an electronic keyboard. The performer added punctuations and carefully timed quiet music throughout the service. The front of the church was actually a raised stage, and the speakers and keyboardist occupied all of it, while Karl's casket, which was closed when the service began, sat a silent participant on the floor below the stage.

I listened to the eulogy, given by John Campbell, but my mind raced with details long put away in the closed places of my psyche. And my performer son, Kurt, sang and played "Amazing Grace," just as he did at my mother's funeral. That pretty much took care of any remaining dry eyes in the church.

Sitting next to me during the funeral service was the great fullback Bill "Boom Boom" Brown and his second wife, who is lovely. Bill spoke in a whisper and seemed distant though friendly (although I am not certain he was completely aware of his surroundings). Bill was hunched over and had very little movement in his neck, so he had to twist his body to speak directly to me. Watching him shuffle when he walked, it was impossible to imagine this suffering man had been one of the hardest hitting running backs in Minnesota Vikings history.

I was also stunned at the shocking physical condition of many other Vikings veterans. They were whispering shadows of their former greatness because they were now bent over, some brain damaged, some from back surgeries, some with replacement knees. Most of them shuffled on canes and crutches. Almost all of them had paid a very heavy physical toll for the privilege of suiting up with the Minnesota Vikings. I remembered them all as larger than life, virile, and vital. Seeing so many of them together once again after thirty-five years brought back a flood of memories.

Jim "Wrong Way" Marshall hobbled over on canes for a brief talk. He had just had knee-replacement surgery but still radiated his old sparkle. Many others told me of their back and hip surgeries.

Some players had fared better. Though they may have had heart attacks, bypass surgery, or diabetes, they appeared clear-headed. John Campbell, Bob "Benchwarmer" Lurtsema, and Milt Sunde fell into this category. And legendary Coach Bud Grant was still blue-eyed steel, firmly in control of his mind and body. It was good to see him again after all these years, and we had a pleasant talk. Our last meeting had been in the emergency room in 1973, with Karl lying newly paralyzed and about to slip into a months-long coma. Tears had flooded Bud's eyes then—and again now. My own bitter tears would fall a few days later when everything finally sank in.

There was the standard Minnesota funeral dinner in the church hall, but I found I couldn't eat more than a few bites. Steady groups of folks came up to me—I enjoyed many, many conversations and hugs. Then it was time for the funeral cortege to go to the cemetery. Kurt and Kory were among the pallbearers. I wondered what they were thinking and feeling. Having a celebrity dad wasn't always the easiest thing for them.

I did not go to the cemetery. Dmitri and I got into our car, like everyone else, but we drove home. I don't like cemeteries and burials. I'd already seen enough loved ones buried, and I wouldn't be able to stand up very long, anyway.

So the storied life of Karl Kassulke was over, to be remembered or not by history. And, as fate goes, I have survived.

Football Wife

Chapter 1

Going Home, Sweet Home

*M*AY 1962: I AM seventeen years old, graduating with my class of 240 from high school in Boone, Iowa, after a high school career of overachieving in music, athletics, and academics. My name is Jan Kathleen Thatcher, and as salutatorian I give a speech and perform a song at the graduation ceremonies. I will continue part time for the summer at my five-year job at a local department store (at forty cents an hour, with good bonuses for sales acumen), my job as a teacher of swimming lessons in the mornings (I am certified as a water safety instructor), my job as a lifeguard at the local pool in the afternoons, and my jobs on Sunday morning playing organ for two different churches. I have a full-ride scholarship to Drake University in Des Moines, Iowa. I could never dream of attending Drake were it not for the scholarship, as my family has no extra money, especially for a private school. I have a music scholarship (I sing and play cello, organ, and piano), but I will double up and do pre-med as well.

During this summer, my longtime on-again-off-again boyfriend Barry, five years older than I, must go away for National Guard training.

Everyone assumes we will marry, but in his absence I begin to date others and discover, for the first time, that I am attractive.

I did have a small clue about this a month earlier when I won second place in a national writing contest, and the headline in the *Boone News Republican* read "Attractive Boone Senior Wins Writing Contest." But the idea that the opposite sex found me attractive had not yet occurred to me because I was very tall (five feet nine inches at ten years old) at a time when petite and blond was the feminine ideal. My classmates never stopped teasing me. Nor had anyone in my classes ever shown any interest in dating me. But now the boys had caught up with me in height.

So after a whirlwind summer, I pack up my small-town Iowa clothes. My parents borrow a car—we could never afford one—and off we go to Des Moines, forty miles away, quite a distance for me to attend my university studies.

After all, another fine university, Iowa State, is only twelve miles from my house, and I have also been offered a scholarship there. My brother, Bruce, graduated from there as well. In Iowa State's Student Union I also witnessed, at the age of fifteen, my first flasher. When the man opened his trench coat and revealed his naked privates, I had broken out laughing. This is not the reason I chose Drake, though.

I wanted to experience the more diverse, geographically and economically, student body at Drake. So when we arrive in Des Moines, my parents and I travel up and down the three flights of stairs at my dorm, Stalnaker (affectionately known as "stark naked"). We carry loads of clothes, a salmon-colored portable Olympus typewriter, my old turquoise-boxed record player and record collection, and a care package of Mom's best cookies. After many tiring trips, I'm finally installed for the school year.

My roommate, Darcy, is already moved in and has claimed her bed. My parents wave a nostalgic good-bye, hug me, and quickly leave, for they must hurry to return the borrowed car. And so I march forward into life.

Like many second-level "Ivy League schools," Drake has a fine curriculum and a student body of mostly eastern private-school kids who didn't make it into Harvard or Yale. I am intimidated, as they've all had much more advanced courses in high school than I, and they are richer and way more sophisticated in manner and dress. But as classes get going, I quickly learn that I am at no disadvantage. I can do as well or better than they.

At Drake I am exploring a whole new world, a world where celebrity children matriculate (Paris Garroway, daughter of television commentator Dave Garroway, is in my dorm) and heirs and heiresses are often the norm, not the exception. In quick succession I date the heir to the Revlon fortune and then the heir to a bank owner's fortune, both from out of state. In fact, I date a different guy nearly every night for about six weeks, so heady is this discovery of my own attractiveness.

I join an elite sorority, Kappa Kappa Gamma, passing whatever muster it is to be admitted through the Greek Rush process. The students in this sorority are wonderful—classic beauties, bright, witty, and obviously going to be rich married women when they finish at the university. Even the current Miss Iowa is in my pledge class.

Most of the required education given by the sorority to the pledgees has to do with proper ladylike comportment. "Never walk while you're smoking," "Hold a cigarette properly," (none of that matters much to me since I don't smoke), and "Cross your legs at the ankle, never at the knee." Certainly, academic standards must be maintained as well—tutors will be provided if necessary—and of course we are expected to focus our dating attentions on fraternity men.

This is a time when girls, as we will be called for the next thirty years, are expected to wear a skirt to classes, and attendance is mandatory. Absences are expected to be explained clearly and must not be for frivolous reasons, since that could result in negative marks.

It is 1962 and more conservative than seems possible in 2010. Elvis Presley is scandalous, most everyone attends church or synagogue weekly, and the Beatles will make history in 1964 by being allowed on *The Ed Sullivan Show.* Until this year, our skirt lengths were no shorter than a mandatory seven inches from the floor, and all the female teenagers and women, no matter how thin, wear girdles to avoid unseemly jiggles. Two-piece swimsuits have been introduced—with about

one inch of flesh showing between the top and the bottom. Television's
Cleaver family leads the way for family values and ideals.

+〜+

I JUMP into classes big-time. I am taking twenty-two credits—the average course load is fifteen—in order to do a double major. I also attend
my jobs as pianist for a modern dance group and busgirl at the cafete-
ria, for I would have no money at all otherwise. I sing in two university
choruses and play cello in the Des Moines symphony. One of my credits is private cello lessons, which require hours alone each day in a
practice room.

And I enthusiastically join any interesting extracurricular possibility that comes along. I am drunk with this new life, although I do not
now, and never will, drink any alcohol, as I wasn't exposed to it in my
family. For many years people will urge me to "just try this one, you'll
like it," but no matter how much sugar and fruit and color were added,
I just don't like the taste of alcohol. I am stubborn on this issue. Why
drink something I don't like?

Drake also has a fine athletic department. They have long been
known for their outstanding spring track festival called the Drake Relays, and right now they also have a stunning football team, thanks to a
senior who transferred to Drake as a junior when his first university,
Marquette in Milwaukee, Wisconsin, dumped their football program.
His name is Karl Kassulke, and he is a phenomenon, scoring tons of
winning points at each game. He's already been voted the most valuable player last year and will be again at the end of this football season.

He's also set the modern record for kickoff returns—ninety-five
yards against Idaho State.

But I am not interested in football—I never had time for a single
game while in high school because I worked on Friday nights. At
Drake, the football men have a club called the D Club. In accordance
with their rules, all freshmen are required to wear a ridiculous blue
beanie (well, really only the girls have to). I will ignore this rule and
never wear the beanie. I have grown up with three older brothers who
didn't much like having a younger sister they had to babysit, so I don't

like being pushed around by the guys. But if the D Club athletes catch you without a beanie, they have a punishment for you.

One day in early October I am caught by three muscular thugs who grasp me tight (this would never be allowed now, since it would be sexual harassment), then use a bright red indelible lipstick to paint a brilliant *D* on my forehead, something like the scarlet letter, I guess. I can see their names on their blue and white Drake Bulldog athletic jackets: Karl, Willie, and Jim. In return for the red *D,* I lash out and land a solid kick on the thigh of the one named Karl, and he shouts, "Goddamn, I'm sure as hell glad I'll never be marrying you!"

The next week all the girls from the different sororities are in the field house preparing for the annual powder puff football game (one quarter of football to precede the homecoming game): the sorority girls against the independents (non-Greek). I have volunteered to be on the sorority team. The captain of the football team, Jim Evangelista, a dark, good-looking Italian guy from Chicago, is coaching the sorority girls. I develop an immediate crush on him, but he isn't especially interested in me. (It will be some time before I understand how tightly different groups of humans stay together in regard to marriage: the rich to the rich, the Italians to the Italians, the Jewish to the Jewish, the Catholics to the Catholics, the private schools to the private schools, and the Greeks to the Greeks.)

This is my first introduction to the rules of football. At this stage in my life, I've never even seen a football game, let alone played in one, so I'm clueless. But I'm tall, thin, and athletic, so I get the prime positions of center and kick returner.

The other team is being coached by Karl Kassulke, who apparently remembers me from the thigh whacking of the previous week and has his eye on me. Though he is coaching the other team, he is watching me. And I see he's *watching* me. He's *really* watching me a lot. Suddenly, right in the middle of the coaching and instructions, Jim Evangelista looks up and hollers out of nowhere: "Hey Karl! Her name is Jan Thatcher."

So along comes the first practice kickoff. I have been instructed to catch the ball and run as far down the field toward our goal as I can. Well, I catch the ball, all right, then I'm immediately knocked down and kicked hard in the right kidney and in the head. I don't think it was done on purpose, but I am aware of great pain in my back and cannot catch my breath. Then I pass out. I am unconscious, so Karl and Jim throw me in their car and truck me off to Methodist Hospital, where it is determined I have a kidney contusion (bright red blood in my urine) and a concussion. I'm admitted to the hospital for four days and miss the powder puff game and the homecoming game and dance, but I am now clearly the object of Karl Kassulke's romantic interest.

Well, he is a handsome devil, with deep blue eyes, black hair, a rugged nose already broken many times, and an infectious signature laugh that is rather like a goose would sound if it were inhaling and honking incessantly at the same time. He is a rogue, daredevil college hero, perpetually happy, and obviously deeply taken with me. He visits me three times a day, bringing flowers and fruits and candies and yummy corned beef sandwiches from the amazing deli just off campus. He makes me laugh by wiggling his two fake front teeth that are on a removable bridge—the result of a kick in the mouth during a football game. This is just the beginning of what I will learn is the physical beating borne by football players.

When it's time for me to be discharged from the hospital, Karl proudly ferries me back to Stalnaker in his '49 Ford (which has no brakes; he must use the hand brake to stop the car, but I'm still sedated and don't feel alarmed). Fortunately, there are few hills between the hospital and the dormitory, so he has little trouble cranking on the emergency brake at each stop sign. It's comical, something I've never seen before. At the dorm, he takes my arm and helps me to my room, vowing he will come back often—which he does. Of course, in these days men are not allowed in the women's dormitory, but getting me to my bed is an exception that's allowed just this once.

From that day on I date only Karl, which requires me to break several important dates for future dances and events on the Greek calendar. This does not please the sorority, but I have decided to give Karl a serious try. He's a hard person not to love. He's kind, funny, attentive, and seemingly unaffected by his fame. At five feet and eleven and a half inches (all the stats books will round it off to six feet) and 195 pounds,

Karl has a spectacular body, strongly muscled in an amazing and natural way, which complements his rugged good looks. And he is noticeably bowlegged, a trait that makes his walk nearly as unique as his laugh. He is so bowlegged, one of the sportswriters for the *Des Moines Register and Tribune* nicknamed him "Cowboy" Kassulke, a name that stuck while he was at Drake.

We are strongly attracted to each other. From the beginning, both our sets of genes are screaming, Get that one! Get that one! And I fall rapidly and completely into infatuation.

So we take to going out every night, but I must be back in the dorm strictly by 10:00 p.m. because the doors are then locked for curfew. For the last fifteen minutes before curfew, all the guys and gals lean against the outside walls of Stalnaker, furiously making out. The smell of raging hormones is in the air. Sighs, smacking, sucking, and various other rutting sounds are clearly heard. The dorm mother is observing all this with great disapproval, but there's nothing she can do about it except keep jangling the keys that will lock the doors at precisely10:00 p.m. I will never once break curfew. There are some rules I'm careful not to break, and this one seems serious. I have no idea how I would get to my room if I were locked out, and a stay overnight in the boys' dorm could get me expelled. Even a visit to Karl's room could result in expulsion, so I never see anything but the outside of the building where Jim and he room together.

Beginning with the very first time Karl and I make out against this wall, he "creams his jeans." I know what this is because girls do talk! I'm very flattered that he finds me so completely beguiling that just my kiss and touch causes him to orgasm. So every night he leaves me and walks stiffly back to his own dorm, and I run up the stairs of the dorm to gossip with friends and maybe do some homework.

By mid-November we're madly in love and determined to marry the following summer, as Karl will clearly be playing pro football somewhere. He wants me to be with him, wherever that is. I'm absolutely confident he will play professional football, though the odds against that are very high (but I do not realize this). So he's proposed to me, and I have accepted. Now we're going to Boone to get my parents' permission.

This will be my first real taste of what celebrity might mean in our lives. Everywhere we go in Boone, people stop us and ask for his autograph and hope to talk with him. It's still football season, and Drake may win the conference. I do notice that Karl is very anxious to please all these fans, sometimes even when it inconveniences our plans.

My own parents go gaga at his presence in our home. When he asks permission to marry me—I am not yet eighteen—my parents give their easy agreement, as long as I promise to finish college. I have every intention of finishing college, and then some. It never once occurs to me that I can't do everything—be married, go to school, and have children like right now, which is expected of all married women. How naive and foolish I am. My own risk taking and leaping without looking will cause me plenty of pain over the years, but lots of good lessons too.

+〜+

AT SEVENTEEN I'm sure I know everything there is to know about life. After all, I'm the only young person I know who's experienced a tragic death in the family; my brother was killed in an auto accident when I was fifteen. And in grade school I was often ill, interacting again and again with doctors and hospitals and sometimes missing as much as a year of school.

My mother was often hospitalized as well, once at bed rest in a full-body cast for six months. During these times I needed to become the chief cook and bottle washer in the family. I developed a love of cooking from all this. My mother was a superb cook, and I learned a great deal from her.

I remember the time she was coming home from the hospital after a monthlong stay, and I decided to bake a mocha chocolate cake from scratch for her. I looked up a recipe in her cookbook. It called for three teaspoons of coffee, but I didn't understand it meant liquid coffee, so I cheerfully dumped three teaspoons of ground coffee into the frosting. It looked stunning.

I couldn't wait for Mom and Dad to taste the special treat when they arrived home from the hospital. When the time came, they each cut a large wedge and dug in. The expressions on their faces changed from pleasure to puzzlement and then polite spitting into their nap-kins. I burst into tears. The day was saved by scraping off the frosting, and I learned a valuable lesson about mocha and reading between the lines in cookbooks.

Cleaning the house during mom's illnesses was another thing. Though she provided me with a good education in cleaning, sewing, and ironing, I took no pleasure in these things. Had they been graded like classes, I would have flunked. Clean clothes, waiting to be ironed, were piled to staggering heights in the laundry room waiting for the water spritzes and a hot iron to make them wearable. Dust curls were gathered in all the corners of the house. Missing buttons had not been replaced, and the mantels would certainly not pass the white glove test. I made up my mind to hire some help when I had my own home, and I would end up doing exactly that for many years.

And I already knew I could handle any financial situation, because money problems were severe in my family. I successfully learned this could be taken care of neatly for my needs if I worked at enough jobs, which I gladly did beginning at age eight. I remember buying my mother a vase for Mother's Day on weekly installments of twenty-five cents earned from delivering *TV Guide* on my bicycle. Each week I had to make the deliveries, then go around at least twice more to try to collect the monies due. I earned eighty cents a week at age eight, and I thought I was on top of the world.

What other kind of trouble can there be to struggle through in life? I am supremely naive and confidant, so Karl and I are officially engaged.

Our next task is to announce this development to his parents, who have no clue that Karl is serious about a girl. So over the Thanksgiving vacation we pack up his old Ford, including my cello, and set off for Milwaukee. I will be meeting Karl's entire family—his parents and his four siblings—for the first time. Karl hasn't talked much about his family, and I haven't paid much attention to this. Who cares about family when you're madly in love?

I am about to learn and witness a great deal of new things, some not so pleasant. But first, we have to get to Milwaukee. We're still driving the

'49 Ford without brakes. It never occurs to me to ask why the brakes aren't just fixed. It's not like Karl is broke. He always seems to have money. I'm just not paying attention to these kinds of details.

At about 1:00 a.m., the Ford stops running for no obvious reason just outside Dubuque, Iowa. There are no cell phones in this era, and we have no idea what to do. My cello is valuable, and I don't want to leave it in the cold, because it could easily crack. We can't just go off down the road without a plan.

Along comes a semitrailer truck, which stops, its brakes loudly huffing in the silent cold while the headlights illuminate our poor car. The driver seems overjoyed at our predicament and offers us shelter for the night at his home in Dubuque. Then he'll help us get the car fixed in the morning. I am with a very strong man, a celebrity who is immediately recognized by the truck driver, so I don't feel at all anxious about this arrangement. So we climb up the steep steps into his cab, pull in the cello, and off we go.

When we arrive at his house, it's 2:00 a.m. We are met at the door by the truck driver's wife, who is wielding a rolling pin above her head and is about to clobber her husband. Her face is screwed into a red map of rage. I thought this was just something to read about in the comic strip *Blondie*. I didn't think it actually happened in real life.

My eyes are about to pop out of my head, but Karl seems surprisingly quiet about this development. In a few days I'll understand better why he does not react much.

The trucker's wife is angry because it seems our good Samaritan had been out catting around. We are his foils; she can't hit him in front of us. So we're grudgingly left to our own devices in the guest bedroom and hold each other tight while we listen for the next two hours to a screaming match that includes several four-letter words I thought were never spoken aloud. Finally all is quiet, though I wonder if everyone will still be alive when we wake in the morning.

I grew up in a family where there was no money, but it was still white collar. Rarely was a voice raised, and there was no drinking and no outward evidence of dysfunction to my seventeen-year-old mind (later life would prove me wrong in this respect too). Right now, just the smallest voice is whispering in the darkest part of my mind, "Maybe you don't know everything."

But true to his word, the fellow helps us get the car going in the morning, and we're back on our way to Milwaukee. There is no mention of the previous night, though I notice several fresh scratch marks on the truck driver's face—rather deep, actually. And Karl is still very cheerful and joking, as if nothing at all happened.

For the rest of the way into Milwaukee, Karl fills me in on his family. The trucker's situation seems to have triggered his need to talk about them. Karl's grandparents on both sides emigrated from Germany. I never actually get the whole story of the reasons for their emigration. The one family story I am told, and will hear repeatedly over the years, is that Grandpa Kassulke had a booming bar business in Milwaukee, and when he died, he did not leave the bar to his eldest son, Karl's dad, Otto, as was expected. Instead, he sold the bar, Karl says, in order to slow down Otto's heavy drinking. The bar was named Kassulke's, of course, but the new owner changed the name.

In the future, whenever Otto bitterly retells this story, everyone in the family looks at their hands and sighs. And interestingly, I will never hear of or meet any other member of either side of Karl's family, except Grandma and Grandpa Freitag, Leona's sweet parents. It's almost as if Otto and Leona (Karl's mom) were the only children in their families, which I know they were not.

Karl continues his story. Otto was grudgingly employed his entire career at the local Harnishfeger factory, a company that made giant mining and construction equipment. But the bile from losing that bar never left Otto's throat and mind. He complained about it daily and drank away his anger every night before coming home to dinner. His favorite drink, Karl explains, is a boilermaker—brandy washed down with beer.

All this talk about alcohol on our way to Milwaukee is also new to me. I had already seen that Karl liked his beer, but I had never seen him drunk or disorderly from it. Nor had I ever seen anyone else in that condition, so I am getting a bit uncomfortable for what Karl seems to be implying.

I am prepared to meet his family: his mother Leona, maiden name Freitag; his older brother Willard, a Lutheran minister; and his three younger sisters, Carmen, Christine, and Kathleen. I'm not prepared for the typical Milwaukee blue-collar home. As we drive up, Karl explains that his family lives in the downstairs "flat." As it applies to housing, *flat* is a new word for me. Another entire family lives upstairs in what seems like a regular-sized house.

When we enter the flat, Leona—a thin, tense, wiry woman—rushes to embrace Karl and welcome me. I quickly learn she is both a very nice lady and also has a hysterical edge to her, particularly in her laugh. No inhaling goose in this laugh. It's a shrill scream, a laugh I've never before heard. It's a mix of laughter and horror, though it is frequent and delivered through a tightly smiling face.

I look about and cannot imagine how so many people can live in this two-bedroom space, but they have it all worked out somehow. I meet Karl's sisters, who clearly adore him. Then Willard stops by. Much taller than Karl, Willard has more of his mother's thin build, and I feel he is appraising me. I'm not necessarily sure he approves, but eventually he will be a strong supporter.

Then the big man arrives home. Otto Kassulke is built like an older Karl, heavily muscled but deeply red in the face and clearly drunk. He's jovial at first and thrilled to see Karl and talk about football—his boy, his pride, his joy in life. Leona is more tense now that Otto's home, as are the girls. He pays very little attention to me for the time being. My time is coming, though.

We finally all sit down for a family dinner, which is still the way things are done in 1962. But this dinner will hold some surprises for me. Otto begins to chat with me. It's in the form of direct questions and statements, delivered while eating and not looking at me.

"Karl tells me you like science."

"Yes," I answer, "I like science."

"So you really like science?"

"Yes," I repeat, "I really like science."

"Do you think you'll be a scientist some day?"

"Maybe," I answer.

"Well," he says, wickedly grinning at his spoon, "I think all scientists are atheists!"

A deep silence falls over the table. This comment was obviously meant as a deep insult to me and as an expression of severe disapproval. I have no idea what to say. I've never heard people speak to each other this way, so I just keep quiet, like everyone else.

We're having corned beef and cabbage for dinner. It's tasty, but the corned beef is a bit undercooked and really tough. All the food is in one pot in the center of the table, so we've been helping ourselves out of this pot.

Suddenly, Otto picks up his plate and, with a dramatic flourish, pours all his half-eaten food back into the pot. Then he says, "This goddamned food is pissant tough, and no pig could even eat it! I'm going to the corner for a few drinks and some decent food."

He stands up. Leona moves near him to try to reason with him. Before I realize what's happening, he smacks her hard in the face with his ham-hock fist. She falls on the floor without a word. No one else says a word either or moves to help Leona. There is no sound at all. Everyone looks away. Otto turns, weaves a bit, and stalks out the door, slamming it behind him with bearish force. In a brief, stunning moment, my whole fairy-tale world turns to a course in Reality 101.

Well, this is sure new stuff. I have no idea how to react, especially since everyone else seems to be ignoring the entire thing. I guess I'd heard about something like this and had seen *A Streetcar Named Desire,* but I had never, ever seen it in real life.

That night Karl tells his mom of our plans to marry the following July. She seems happy, then disappears into her room. She returns with a very small, yellowish diamond ring without sparkle. She proudly presses it into my hand and says, "This was my mother's wedding ring, now it will be yours." I don't know what to say. I'm already wearing the diamond engagement ring Karl and I picked out together, and the matching wedding band is nestled in a box in one of Karl's drawers back at Drake.

I'm picking up on the idea of how controlling people is part of the rules in this house. I don't like to be controlled. I was often called willful while I was growing up. So I decide right then that I will not accept this ring. I very politely return it to Leona, show her my diamond, find the right words, and tell her, "This is something I'm sure you will want to save for your daughter when she marries. But thank you so much for the lovely thought."

Leona appears to be crushed. I know, and I'm truly sorry for her. But it's also clear to me that my refusal of this ring is the least of her problems.

Karl and I pass the rest of the trip to Milwaukee in much the same way. During the day he shows me the sights of his hometown and basks in the glory of his celebrity everywhere he goes. At dinnertime I continue to get acquainted with his family. Everyone is on edge every night, on red alert for another of Otto's obviously frequent fits of violence and anger. I also get my first exposure to bars. Karl knows them all, and they all know him. Everyone appears quite jolly, and everyone seems to have little else to do each evening but sit and drink Milwaukee's famous beer.

We get through the Thanksgiving dinner. I have my eighteenth birthday, and then it's finally time to return to Drake. We don't speak much for the first half of the trip. I have a lot to digest, and I try to understand. It's beginning to dawn on me that I might not really know everything about life. It hasn't yet occurred to me that the scene and events Karl grew up with are going to affect me.

Chapter 2

Preparing for Big Changes

WE RELAX BACK INTO the hectic cocoon of college life. All doors are open to the hero and his campus sweetheart, and life is moment-to-moment honey. We're just a few weeks from the end of the football season now, which will mean the end of Karl's college playing career. The semester will end immediately after that, which means Karl will go to Montgomery, Alabama, to play in the postseason Blue-Gray Football Classic, which is a huge honor.

For now, I will go home for the Christmas holidays and watch Karl's game on national television. After the Christmas vacation, the pro football draft will occur, and everyone seems to feel Karl is guaranteed a try on some pro team. He will find out for sure once this draft happens. So I quickly learn the basic rules for the game of football and the whens, hows, and whys for each particular type of offensive and defensive maneuver so I can talk a good game when questioned.

Meanwhile, there are things to get done before Christmas. We continue seeing each other nightly, and Karl begins teaching me to play cribbage, a card game critical in his life and the life of his family and friends. It requires a wooden peg board, luck, and technique, and he has several fun rhymes he spouts with each particular move: "Fifteen two, fifteen four, that's all, there ain't no more," "Fifteen two, fifteen four, fifteen six, and a pair makes eight" (not a rhyme, but delivered in a singsong style), and "Cut 'em thin to win, deep to weep." All the counting's done rhythmically and is half the fun of the game.

Karl's sneaky about his teaching. In order to keep winning, he doesn't reveal all the rules or techniques at once. I must discover them one by one as he clobbers me again and again. But over the next three weeks, I watch carefully for all the rules he leaves out of my instructions until I finally learn all the tricks. The first time I win, I do a "double skunk," which means Karl basically scored very little before I beat him. Karl looks away for a moment, and I think he's going to be angry, but after a deep breath, he looks back at me and honks a deep laugh my way. "Well, Janny, it looks like you're going to be a tough cribbage player. We'll see if you can keep it up." We'll play thousands of rowdy games of cribbage together over the next ten years—all in fun, jousting back and forth for the win.

Then there's the problem of money. My membership in the sorority is expensive, and my two jobs don't quite cover what I need. So because of my own needs, I now learn about the underworld of finance for college sports stars. I'd wondered where Karl and the other guys received a seemingly endless flow of money for their needs. Everyone knows collegiate rules prohibit giving money, or incentive pay, to star athletes. Yet all the guys seem to have plenty of money without obvious jobs. I have no idea where this money came from until one day Karl announces he must shovel the snow from the sidewalk for a prominent and kind businessman in Des Moines. I'm totally puzzled by this. Who is this man and why did this request come suddenly from someone I'd never met?

It's time for me to learn about the Drake Boosters Club. It is apparently perfectly legal to pay college sports stars if they're working for you. To ensure the ability to entice good players to the school, the men of the Drake Boosters Club made sure there was a way to get money to the players. So Karl shovels thirty feet of sidewalk in ten minutes and gets paid four hundred dollars. This is how it works for all the players on the team. When they need some funds, they do a brief job for a Drake booster—like raking a front lawn or shoveling snow or painting a small fence—and are paid outrageously for the task.

Now I need funds, so I benefit from the Drake Booster's Club too. A kind man pulls some strings for me, and I'm given a plum job as a clerk in the just-off-campus music store. The pay is great, and I can come in when I wish. I feel like a kid in a candy store amongst all that delicious sheet music. With my other two jobs, I now have enough extra money for the rest of the school year.

But the sorority is another issue. I see that belonging to it is draining my funds, and it is probably a needless expense. So though I very much like all my sisters there, I decide to withdraw just before I go home for Christmas. It's bittersweet, because there's a lovely ceremony for all the newly engaged women at the end of each semester, and Karl and I have kept our engagement secret on campus so that I can participate.

On the appointed night of the ceremony, with the darkened grand old room lit by candlelight, all the sorority women sit in a tight circle and await the surprise announcements, which will come, for the most part, from juniors and seniors. The ritual is one of absolute silence, with the suspense building because everyone knows there will be at least one person in the room who will jump into the center of the circle and flash a diamond on her fourth finger, left hand. Until that happens, everyone covers her left hand with her right hand. No one can see the rings. When the newly engaged sister is revealed, everyone hugs her, screams their delight, and then sits down to await any further surprises.

The room and setting are quite romantic, and I'm enjoying the evening. There have been two announcements, and it's been a while since the last. All is expectant hush. Just as the president moves to end the ceremony, I jump into the middle and flash my ring. The room explodes with wows and yahs and just plain screams of joy. They can't believe my good fortune at snagging the college hero (although not a Greek)—and me a freshman yet! The congratulations and hugs go on joyfully for quite a while. Later, over tea and cookies, I take my sorority sponsor aside and tell her I must leave the sorority pledge class now and will not be returning. We both weep, because these are genuinely

special people, and I'll miss their camaraderie. But I explain I must prepare for a wedding, and it will take all my extra funds.

After this event, I rarely see any of my sorority friends. The rule
about Greek and independents not mixing holds, and I'm not invited
to their events. We move off into separate worlds, except for my Kappa
friend Pat, who is from Minneapolis. She doesn't return to Drake for
her sophomore year because she got married. She will remain my lifelong friend in Minneapolis.

Then, there's the sex. Karl and I have not yet been going all the
way, but it's clear things are headed in this direction. I've already decided not to worry about pregnancy; we'll be married in seven
months, anyway. So in a cold, cramped car just before the end of
exams and the semester, we finally do the deed. Stuffed in the unfor-
giving front seat of an old stick-shift car, we fumble around and get
the windows completely steamed. We neck and pet, and suddenly he
urgently says, "Now, now, hurry!"

I'm happy to hurry. It's darn cold without my clothes on, and I'm
really nervous about getting caught. We don't use birth control. I find
pleasure in the intimacy, soft kisses, gentle caresses, and lovemaking,
especially the feeling of being completely treasured and living in a perfect body. But we have to be on the lookout for the police banging their
flashlights on the steamed windows of parked cars or teenagers prank-
ing about doing the same thing. So there is also an unpleasant tension.

We just finish dressing when the flashlight banging starts. The light
explores the entire interior of the car and both of us. "Oh, no problem,
officer, we'll be leaving right away."

Then, with final exams successfully over (I've managed to maintain
an A- average in order to keep my scholarship, despite my less-than ad-
mirable study habits), we part for the Christmas season. I catch a ride
home with another Drake student who lives in Boone, and Karl heads
to Milwaukee in his brakeless Ford.

⁺◦⁺

ENTERING MY family home is like going into a Christmas fairyland. Every
open space is covered with red, white, and green decorations, crèches,

homemade chains and crocheted decorations on the tree, and miniature Christmas villages. The holidays at my house were always short on presents and long on loving, cooking, and family fun. So we sing around the piano, gorge ourselves on Mom's famous cookies decorated like miniature pieces of art, down meals of amazing taste, have friends over, and go visiting. Of course, there's singing in the church choir for the Christmas special events and some organ playing to be done. The climax of the holiday is the Christmas Eve service, with the manger scene in the candlelit church, the low lighting, the endless carol singing, and finally, the three wise men parading down the center aisle in their theatrical finery.

After church we have a four-star home dinner and then open our gifts, following our usual fun ritual. My mother has written a poem on each gift tag, and each package is elaborately and lovingly wrapped. The point of the poem is to be a clue about what is in the package. The recipient must try to guess what the gift is before opening. So Mom and Dad, my two remaining brothers, Bruce's wife and daughter Shon, and Jerry's two foster sons, and I sit in a circle and open our gifts one at a time, waiting until each present is carefully unwrapped (to save the paper) and enjoyed by all before the next gift is opened. Even with a few gifts, we are at this game until well after midnight.

Finally, the big day arrives. Not Christmas, but the Blue-Gray game at Montgomery, Alabama. Karl is the starting offensive halfback, so we'll see a lot of action from him. My family and I gather around the big television console (black-and-white screen, of course). Excitement and tension run high in the room. I'm so proud that my future husband will probably be the star of the game. Not everyone in the room is interested in football, but we all stare at the screen, watching for Karl's jersey number.

He receives the kickoff and makes a nice return. He carries the ball several times for great runs. He's doing his usual magic, fearlessly plowing straight ahead, often against much bigger men. Then suddenly he is tackled, and something is clearly terribly wrong. He doesn't get up, but writhes on the ground in pain. The coach runs out to see what's going on. He motions for other help. Soon Karl is on a stretcher being carried out, and that's the end of his Blue-Gray game.

We strain at every word from the announcer as they prognosticate. "Maybe it's a head injury... The great Karl Kassulke is down... Will he be back?... Yes, folks, he's the hardest hitting running back in the college ranks... Tragic possible loss..." But no one seems to know what has actually happened. This is my first of many anxious waits to hear what the injuries are and how serious they are. Will his football career be over? Will he survive? Will the damage be permanent? There is nothing to do but wait and worry.

All is silent in the room as the television announcers run their mouths. All eyes are on me. I must remain calm. I must be brave, and now I see that to be a football wife will mean many of these scenes. Television cameras will find me in the crowd and focus on my reaction while my husband's fate is in limbo. Finally we hear he's been taken to the hospital with an arm injury.

It's eight hours later when he calls me with devastating news. He has finally come out of anesthesia after the repair of a shattered right forearm (at least he's left-handed!). Both bones have been broken in a total of six places. He has two metal plates and eight screws holding the mess together, and of course a full arm cast. The pain is terrible. He says the doctor told him he will never play again, but then he says, "That's bullshit! I'll get this cast off and be as good as new. Nothing will stop me from playing!" This proves to be true. Eight weeks later he's out of the cast as if nothing happened.

A few days after Christmas, I take a train to Milwaukee to be with Karl. He's up and about and jolly, seemingly pain-free. He's making the rounds of the bars, happy to see me and playing his beloved cribbage. His family is more tense than ever, though no one speaks of his injury. There is some new tension I don't understand over a parking ticket Karl ignored. And Leona hits the kitchen floor once again while I'm there (and then sports an appalling black eye for the rest of our visit). A few years later Otto will try to physically bully me, which doesn't work out very well for him, and I do see him slug Karl once, but it looks like Leona is on the receiving end of most of the violence. About now I'm wondering who put the "fun" in "dysfunctional." And though I don't yet know the word for it, I am receiving a strong lesson in denial.

WE GET back to Drake after the traumatic holidays. I'm taking twenty-two credits again, plus the other extras, and working three jobs. Karl isn't playing football now, so he has even more time to be with me. One day I mention to Karl I'm fatigued. I'm keeping a grueling schedule, so fatigue would be quite natural. His response is, "No problem, just come with me to the team physician." This is a doctor with a private practice in Des Moines. When Karl shows up, arm still in a cast and me on the other arm, the doctor is delighted. They talk football and Karl's prospects for the upcoming draft.

Then the conversation turns to my fatigue. The doctor hears all about my schedule, but he does not examine me in any way, then promptly writes me a perpetually renewable prescription—for amphetamines. I'm to take one a day, and the doctor promises I'll have more energy. These amphetamines, little black and white capsules, are a common prescription at this time—way too common. It is years before the full addictive and potential health problems of these drugs are made public. For now, this is a totally normal prescription, and the doctor warns me not to take more than one a day. For the next nine years, I will be taking that one great little pill every day. I never took more than that, but I sure did appreciate the energy that little sucker gave me. The team physicians first prescribed it, then my obstetrician did the same, right through both of my pregnancies.

As a physician in 2010, I am horrified at the idea of a pregnant woman taking amphetamines, but at least two generations of babies were born to moms on this drug. We don't know much about the effect of one pill a day. Addicted moms, though, delivered underweight babies who had to go through withdrawal and suffered learning defects for much of their lives. As another indicator of how little we knew in the 60s and 70s, I was to learn to arrest premature labor with the use of an alcohol drip, and some moms would be on this drip for months before their babies were born. Now we know that even small amounts of alcohol can cause permanent adverse effects on the fetus.

I'm also learning for the first time about the university's system of tutors for the athletes. Karl is smart but not especially ambitious as far as studies go. So one day he leaves me earlier than usual because he has an appointment with his tutor. It seems he hadn't been able to take a full load of classes because of football, and now he doesn't have enough credits to graduate. I didn't know about this. They're going to try to get him through two extra history classes, plus his regular load, which includes student teaching this semester.

Karl's a history major, so he has to have these classes in order to graduate and be a history teacher. Karl's actually not the least bit interested in history or teaching, although he's wildly popular as a student teacher. He's just taking history because someone told him it would be an easy course to get through with his sports. He's not thrilled about this extra study and finally quits those two classes, saying he'll just take them in summer school.

The big talk this final semester is about the pro football draft. There are basically three professional football leagues at this time: the National League, which is considered the premiere league; the American League, the new kid on the block and not quite as premiere; and the Canadian league for the leftovers from the two U.S. professional leagues. A football player's highest hopes at this time are to play in the National League. The Canadian league is better than nothing, but it's a bit embarrassing and offers much less money.

Karl is not the only football player at Drake likely to be drafted, but as the draft day gets closer, more speculative articles about Karl appear in the Des Moines press. Karl keeps quiet about his hopes, but I know he'll be crushed if he isn't drafted by one of the two main leagues. Again, I naively assume he will not only be drafted but will make the team, not realizing that only one or two players out of every hundred drafted actually make a team, and about one player in ten thousand is even drafted in the first place.

Then the big day comes: the National League draft. The first round goes by. Karl isn't chosen, but he didn't really expect to be in the first round. The second, third, and fourth rounds go by without a mention. Then, in the eleventh round, on draft pick number 152, Karl is chosen! A great cheer goes up in the bar where we are watching the draft picks come up on the screen. Karl has been drafted by the Detroit Lions of the National Football League to play as a defensive halfback.

This totally confuses me. For four years he's been starring as an offensive halfback and racking up record points for his teams. Why would they choose him to be a defensive halfback? This is definitely a less glorious position, but Karl takes it in stride. He's just grateful to be drafted. I will never know the reason for the league's decision. I can only guess it has something to do with his relatively small size, but I really don't know, and Karl never mentions it.

Now Karl and the boys start to party in earnest. Two other players from the team have been drafted as well, so the drinking is on. Quarterback Terry Zang was drafted by the Green Bay Packers (and would stick for a few years as the backup to the great Bart Starr), and guard Jerry Bartol was drafted by the Los Angeles Rams (but he doesn't seem to have made the team). We're all excited beyond words, but beer evidently expresses it well. The drinking age is twenty-one, but I never once see any of the bars around Drake checking any IDs. I guess it's a good thing they don't. What on earth would these guys do for celebration if not for beer?

I have to leave around 9:00 p.m. to study for a test the next day, so I kiss Karl good-bye, wave to the boys at the bar, and walk back to my dorm. They're all so full of good cheer, they barely notice my leave-taking.

The next morning I see Karl after my exam is over. He's still very, very drunk, and I have never seen him like this. I don't like it at all. I don't understand his behavior and have no patience with his silliness. The more I ask him to straighten out, the worse he gets. Things escalate gradually and steadily until I am thoroughly angry. I can't figure out why he would just keep behaving this way.

We are now having our first major fight, and I am discovering that there is no way to fight with a drunk. They aren't going to be logical and linear; they're full of silly, sloppy, slobbering nonsense.

"Whas amatter, Janny? Aren't you happy for me? Oh, just a

minute... I've gotta piss." And he moves tight to the building and does just that.

I'm finally so frightened and fed up with his behavior, I take off my ring, throw it at him, and stalk off. I know I don't want to live with something like this in my house!

The next day he catches up with me on the way to one of my classes and begs my forgiveness. He just got overexcited with his draft pick. "It will never, never happen again. Please, please take the ring back, Janny. You're my Janny-Bananny. Come on, let's make up. It will never happen again. I'm sorry. I'm really sorry."

Well, I'd never seen him drunk before (though to be truthful, I had heard rumors about his drinking), so I take the ring back and believe him when he makes these promises, because I want to believe him. And I never do see him drunk again—until after we're married.

One of the other decisions I make concerns my choice of career. I love music and have been getting A's in all my studies. I have a fortunate ability to sight-read the most complicated music and also have perfect pitch (not in my singing, but in knowing what note is being played). I know I am no genius, and it's clear to me that if I continue in music, I will have a career as a music teacher (which I don't want). I will not have a career as a performing musician.

I discover two important things at Drake: first, gifted musicians are a dime a dozen, and second, I really don't like to spend hours alone in the practice rooms each day. So I make the correct decision that music will be my avocation, a lifelong pleasure, and science will be my career. I decide I'll be a doctor, though everyone I speak to insists I must be a nurse. Women just don't go to medical school at this time. Karl makes no comment either way. Right now he isn't worrying about my career.

·~·

BEFORE THE semester ends, I have some more fun with Karl's old black Ford. I'm taking eastern saddle riding for my physical education class, and the stable is several miles off campus. Getting there is never a problem, since there is a several-blocks-long hill to get up, and the emergency brake is rarely needed. But coming back to Drake, I must come down that hill. It reminds me of our sledding days as kids, when we whizzed through street intersections without a thought to danger. That is what this car trip feels like twice a week.

At the very end of the semester, in my last trip down the hill, acrid smoke fills the car, as usual, with me yanking on the emergency brake with all my might. Just as I approach the last intersection, I see another car coming from the left. If it's going the usual speed, I'll get by without a problem. Just then, there's a mighty snap, and I'm suddenly holding the emergency brake handle in my hand with some cable attached—and the car is just going merrily on through the intersection. I'm not aware that I could try to throw the car into reverse and stop it. Of course, the engine would fall out too. But I don't know any of this.

Instead, I can see the eyes of the other driver, a young man, widen as he sees he is going to hit me. He swerves dramatically into some bushes instead, where his car stops abruptly. I speed on through the intersection and can't slow down for another several blocks. Once I have slowed down, I situate the car near the curb and creep the rest of the way to Drake in first gear at five miles an hour.

"Karl, dammit, get those brakes fixed!" I yell when I see him. "Somebody's going to get killed!"

"Okay, Janny, I'll get them fixed. Honk, honk!" So he has the brakes fixed the next day.

The rest of the school year passes in a blur. It's capped by the Drake Relays. The D Club chooses a sweetheart for their queen to ride in the gigantic relays parade. I'm nominated (my first and only beauty queen nomination), Miss Iowa is nominated, and the third nominee is a cute little blonde who has been engaged for three years to another football player. She wins, and I am the runner-up. But we all three ride on the back of a convertible in the parade, waving and having a fine time on a bright spring day. It's sure a new feeling for me.

I'm jolted during this parade, though, to see my old boyfriend for the first time since he left for the National Guard. Barry had, of course, received my "Dear John" letter while he was away at training. He's standing on the sidewalk along the parade route, looking sad, together with some of our friends from that time. We wave, and I pass on by.

The academic year is dwindling, with just a few days left. When I stop long enough to reflect on all the newness and strangeness, joys and uncertainties, and finalities of this year, it's almost overwhelming. I'll no longer be a teenager, no longer exploring the world as a single person.

Mostly, though, I don't stop to think. I just keep steaming straight ahead. There's so much to do. I have to finish my finals and term papers, say good-byes to my friends (most of whom I'll never see again, and I sense that and feel a loss), plan a wedding on a dime, arrange Karl's summer school, arrange a job for me that will support us both for a few months, and get accepted and registered for the fall quarter at Wayne State University in Detroit. And then it's over. That's that. At eighteen I'm moving into the real adult world of married life and celebrity.

And so, with sadness, Karl and I drive away from Drake University, a place of great discovery that has changed our lives forever. In a finely tuned and brake-able car, we chat on the forty-mile trip to Boone. We'll be making this trip many times over the summer, but somehow this feels like the end.

Karl senses my melancholy. He takes my hand in his (though I have to then move with the stick shift) and says, "Janny, the world is ours. We're going to have adventure and travel. I'm going to be famous, and I'll be so proud to have you as my wife by my side. Life is just swell! Honk, honk, honk," as he laughs with little boy glee.

I will not attend school at Drake again, but the school alumni association doesn't ever forget me when it's time for the yearly fund drive.

◆◆◆◆◆◆◆◆◆◆◆◆◆◆

Chapter 3

The Long, Strange Summer

*J*UNE 1, 1963: Karl is staying in the office/spare bedroom at my Boone home until our wedding. His bed is screened off from the house by a freestanding bamboo screen. This is the home of my mother's dreams: a Frank Lloyd Wright design lovingly built by a local contractor. It's quite small, with only one bathroom, no basement, and two bedrooms. But it's fitted with special built-ins and nooks throughout the mostly wood interior. The long living room is two solid walls of windows and pegged wood floor.

Our yard, however, is very large, with a mammoth, graceful weeping willow tree shading the back of the house and a working pump well in the backyard that spouts cold, pure water. Mulberry trees are thick with juicy purple-staining fruit, apple and plum trees flower, and the grass, growing in thick, black peat, is so luxurious it's like walking on a cushioned carpet. Living among all this beauty for the past five years will influence my choice of home styles and sites for the rest of my life.

Karl settles in. I'm sure this feels very different from the Milwaukee flat he's used to, and the life of a family of nondrinkers will be very strange for him indeed. But one of his easy traits is his unquestioning flexibility. He's happy to go along with whatever's happening, clearly wishing, above all, to please those people for whom he cares. This will not always be a good thing later in his life.

For instance, though he has grown up in a strong Lutheran environment and has a Lutheran minister brother, he joins my Methodist church without any discussion or argument. And though my family is Republican, I've already decided to be a Democrat, and Karl immediately makes the same decision and even appears at Democratic fund-raisers during our marriage. After our divorce, he will once again change political sides, becoming a very conservative Republican in accordance with the belief system of his new family. These are all perfectly fine decisions, but many things he will do in the future—going along with friends, players, and fans—will be increasingly self-destructive.

For now, we begin a hectic routine. We have much to do in the five weeks before our wedding on July 7, 1963, at the Boone First Methodist Church. Most of the planning is already done. All the invitations are sent, the seamstress sewing my dress is finished—she's also created a sweet blue jacket and sheath dress for my honeymoon trousseau—the attendants are all chosen and arranged, I've purchased just the right black sexy peignoir, the church and minister are reserved, and the organist and soloists are prepared. The wedding ceremony will be performed jointly by our Methodist minister and Karl's proud Lutheran minister brother, Willard.

The wedding is the event of the summer in Boone, and my mother will see that it is very special, foodwise. The reception will be at our house, and there will be no alcohol served. This is a big problem for the Kassulke side of the family. Whoever heard of having a wedding without getting drunk and wild partying? They go ahead and plan a bash for after the reception, which I am supposed to know nothing about. The plan is for all the revelers to go to a reserved hall after we have left for our big honeymoon in a sleazy motel in Des Moines. So while my mother busies herself with handmade candies and mints, handmade gifts for the wedding party, menu plans, and seating arrangements, Karl and I finish some of his required classwork so he can graduate.

Every day we travel to Des Moines. He deposits me at my job with the Cargill Company, where I spend my days accounting for bushels of soybeans. It's boring work, but it pays well, and we have gas money and funds for our other needs. Karl is taking just one class per summer session because the course work is very concentrated, so he hangs out on campus at Drake, supposedly studying while I work. When I'm done, we go home and spend most nights studying. Karl is not much interested in these classes, though they are about history, so I find I have to push him to read and remember his course work and really drill him before exams. And writing his papers falls to me. Basically, I'm unexpectedly taking the courses for him, and history is not a favorite for me, though it will become a pleasure in later years.

AT THE end of the first summer session, it's time for the wedding. The day arrives hot and muggy, and the flowing hairdo I wore for the wedding portrait gets trashed as my hair curls and kinks with the humidity. I end up just twisting it up into a cooler style and go with that. We don't spend any money or time with professional makeup artists or hair stylists, as I don't wear much makeup anyway.

There's already been a disaster in the morning before the wedding. My mother sent my father to pick up eight freshly killed chickens she'll use to make her famous fried chicken for the reception. But when dad brings them home, they haven't been cleaned, and suddenly a red alert goes out. We're all called to the kitchen, where we sit pulling feathers and guts off these birds—on the day of my wedding! The room is a fluffy, bloody mess when we're done. Everyone is behind schedule, and I sense the anxiety in my mother that all must be perfect.

I am strangely calm this entire day, as if I'm watching someone else get married. I am detached, realize it, and wonder why. I don't worry about the schedule or the chickens or my hair. I've heard plenty of rumors of the secret second reception planned by Jim Evangelista, Karl's best man, but I don't care. Somehow everything seems like something I just have to get through before beginning the next stage of my life, and in some ways it seems like a big nuisance. I realize no part of these wedding plans are intended to fit my wishes, though my mother would dearly love for me to be more engaged in the process. We're all simply following society's expected norms. I'm trying to please my mom and dad—I am the much-waited-for, much-loved only daughter—but if left to my own decisions, I would prefer to elope and avoid all the people, the handshaking, and the fawning over Karl (which I'm beginning to see I better get used to).

Everything goes completely smoothly at the wedding, and it is beautiful. At the reception at my home afterward, the food is spectacular, as only my mother would do.

Then Mom approaches Karl and says, "Would you get Mrs. Kassulke and begin the line of serving?" Karl promptly finds his mother and steers her to the front of the line, and everyone howls. He hadn't thought of me as "Mrs. Kassulke."

Now it's time for me to change and, amid the rice shower, depart with Karl in our trusty black Ford as we head off for two days of relaxation in Des Moines. I'm all packed and ready to go, but when I open my suitcase to put on the little blue suit so lovingly created for this occasion, I find my brother Bruce has played a little trick.

He wanted to fill my suitcase with rice as a joke, but he didn't have any. So he filled it with oats—I guess he picked them up when he got the chickens. Unfortunately, oats have a tiny bit of oil in them, so my lovely blue suit is now completely dotted with oil stains. I thank him sarcastically for the great joke and decide to wear the suit anyway. It will be the only time I can wear it, since it's ruined. I don't really care. I'm still strangely indifferent to the celebrations and just want to get out of there. It's the first time I realize I'm probably a major introvert pretending to be an extrovert in the world, and I prefer my own company over a crowd or fuss. (Oh, yes, I've learned a lot in freshman psychology!) This desire to avoid big parties and celebrations as much as possible will not serve me well as the wife of a celebrity.

Our honeymoon is uneventful. The motel is squalid, but it is all we can afford. Karl ceremoniously carries me over the room's threshold, and we laugh at the ridiculous scene. The walls are paper thin, and the roaches scuttle at night (something new for me). We finally get real time alone in bed for lovemaking, and I discover that "hurry, hurry!" really is all there is. It will be years before there is therapy for men with premature ejaculation, and many more years before there are medications to simply and efficiently treat the problem. So that's that.

We go to the local amusement park and eat out a few times, once at a really special steakhouse. We are great company for each other. We play cribbage a lot and laugh a lot. Then the two-day honeymoon is over, and we motor back to Boone as the new Mr. and Mrs. Kassulke.

Now we move temporarily into a weekly rental apartment in Boone, which also turns out to be seedy, another thing I'm not used to. It's a regular house, with the upstairs divided into two apartments separated by a hall. It's situated on the main highway that goes right through Boone, so trucks rumble everything in the room every few seconds.

The Iowa summer is roasting hot, and we have no air-conditioning and no breeze comes though the tiny crack that the creaky windows will open. I can smell every meal being cooked in this place, and I'm not impressed. In our own kitchen, I can see the remains of countless such meals stuck on the cooktop backsplash, and I am unable to successfully scrub any of the greasy mess off.

When I'm there alone, the very unkempt man across the hall who wears a stereotypical dirty, sweaty spaghetti-strap T-shirt, repeatedly attempts to molest me. I actually keep a frying pan by the door for when he tries to get in. Even when he doesn't manage to get his hands on me or slap me on the butt, his eyes are so filled with lust that he creeps me out.

He seems to be a bit slow in his thought process, as Karl has strongly informed him of dire consequences if he doesn't leave me alone, but I must endure his leering presence and suggestive remarks every time I go out of my door. He sits in the hall and waits for me to come out, and so I do my best to avoid any trips when Karl isn't around. I feel trapped and irritable.

I'm still working for Cargill in Des Moines, and Karl is finishing the second history class so he can graduate. We settle into another round of tutoring, badgering, paper writing, and cramming for tests. At last, by the end of July, the course is over, and Karl graduates. We will be moving on big-time.

+~+

NOW THE action starts! It's time for Karl to go to the Lions training camp in Deerfield, Michigan, which, like all pro football camps, fills all of August and part of September, breaking up just before the actual football season starts. Wives are not allowed at the camp—the operative word here and everywhere in pro football is *wives*, not *women*. Even so, we newlyweds want to be as close as possible to each other, and I'm still completely naive and confident and assume that Karl, because of his huge talent, will make it with the team.

So we pack all our worldly belongings (mostly wedding presents) into the smallest U-Haul trailer we can rent and head for Detroit. I know nothing about big cities (I've been to Chicago often as a child, but usually under the protective umbrella of relatives). As soon as we arrive in Detroit, I drive Karl to the exclusive suburb of Deerfield, see the training camp quarters, and drop him off. I will not be allowed to see him again during training camp, except for once a week on family days and after the preseason football games. During those family day visits, I notice there are an awful lot of nonfamily beautiful women around who seem to know the players quite well.

I'm eighteen, newly married, a small-town girl, and completely on my own in this dirty, crowded, noisy big city. And I have very little money. Karl doesn't have any money either, as the training camp income is something like a hundred dollars a week, which I quickly learn evaporates from Karl's wallet as fast as he gets it. It will be a while before I learn that Karl tends to, quite literally, piss his money away by drinking gallons of beer. And even years later, at his funeral, I will learn he was part of an ongoing locker room gambling game. I never had any idea about that at the time.

For now, I must immediately get an apartment, one that doesn't require a deposit. So I move into a high-rise with no elevator in inner-city Detroit. The apartment is on the tenth floor, with no air-conditioning and even more roaches than our honeymoon motel. I carry all our belongings up those ten flights of stairs. No one offers any help.

I have to get a job immediately or I will starve. In the next block I discover a storefront temporary work agency: Kelly Girls. They have a job for me as a temporary executive assistant for one of the General Motors executives. I will earn just enough for rent and maybe five dollars a week for food.

I spend my days driving to work, then sitting at a receptionist desk in a plush office, filling in for the vacationing executive assistant. The work is manageable, but this executive world in 1963 is something new for me to navigate. Sexual innuendo, suggestive body rubbing, and overt grabbing seem to be the main reason I'm there. My receptionist and secretarial skills are fine, but no one really seems to care about them. I feel like I'm playing dodge ball all day long if I venture from behind my desk—which I must do.

At night I have a few moments to chat by phone with Karl. Apparently his calls are limited too, for these talks are short and hurried, but at least I can get caught up on his progress. I learn he is being placed at defensive halfback, behind a legendary defensive back named Dick "Night Train" Lane. Apparently Detroit drafted Karl because Night Train was injured earlier in the year and was doubtful for the upcoming season. But now Night Train is back at full tilt, and Karl doesn't think his chances of making the team are very good. I refuse to believe this and keep assuming we're going to live in Detroit, which has certainly underwhelmed me so far as a desirable place.

I don't have enough money to buy food, so I take to cooking plain spaghetti for all my meals. Karl saves a little food for me from the training tables (mostly bread, apples, and oranges), which groan with food for these big men. So once a week for three weeks, I see Karl and get a bit of food to eat. But it isn't enough. By the end of the third week, I am sick with a kidney infection. Karl gets permission from the coach for me to see the team physician, who gives me the wrong medicine, and I am sick for nearly a month with this serious infection.

After three weeks, I'm on the verge of adjusting to this life of work and deprivation and starvation: no television, no radio, no newspapers, no magazines, no books, just the entertaining folks of my apartment complex. They get loud especially at night, with all windows open, and I'm treated to more new slices of life.

Each night, with my single-bulb ceiling light turned off, I position myself by the open window for the slight breeze and listen—and even sometimes see—dramas upon dramas in the other windows up and down the quadrangle of buildings. "If you put your fucking hand on my leg one more time, old man, I'll cut your nuts off," screams a daughter at her dad. "Listen, shitface, I saw you with that whore yesterday, and I'll fuckin' pull her eyes out if I ever catch her around here again!" So many sweet family scenes. These colorful dialogues, punctuated with screams and crying and whacks, last long into the night every night. So who needs television?

I wonder if there's any happiness in this part of the world. If there is, it's quiet. Unhappiness is very loud and up front.

Then, one day after work, Karl calls at his usual time. "Janny, the Lions cut me," he says, and my frazzled spirits are flushed right down the toilet. "And I was picked up by the Minnesota Vikings. I'm already training with them in Portland, Oregon."

Years later, when I read Karl's book, I will discover that Karl was cut after a period of truly brutal hazing. When he finally got mad and injured one of the Lions regulars, the team paid him back with two broken teeth, two black eyes, a broken nose, and several cuts and bruises. I never knew about any of this, and when I saw him again, several weeks later, he had healed from all those wounds. He never said a word about the hazing to me.

With this phone call from Portland, the idea of life turning with the speed of an arrow occurs to me. Here I am in Detroit, eighteen years old, living in a rathole, starving, sick, enduring a crappy job, and my husband is suddenly in Oregon. From there he'll go to the Vikings training camp in Bemidji, Minnesota, at least until mid-September or until he is cut by the Vikings.

I waste no time in renting a U-Haul, quitting my job, forgetting about school at Wayne State University, and clearing out of that apartment. I very carefully shake out my clothes and spray various poisons into all the containers to avoid taking roaches home to Boone. By late afternoon the next day, I'm driving back to my parents' home, relieved that I'll at least get some food and some decent medicine for my tormenting kidney infection. I've been running a fever for three weeks now, and my urine smells dreadful. My only fond memory of Detroit is Vernor's ginger ale, a specialty of the area made from a recipe that's over a hundred years old. Yummy and terrific. But that's it. I'm really glad to get out of that city.

With a few weeks left of training camp, I finally have a short vacation—no job and no studies. The Vikings are a new NFL team. The upcoming season will be their third, and the first two seasons were miserable, with just a few wins. It's still unclear if Karl will make the team. I'm not quite so idealistic now. I sleep a lot and watch the news for the latest rounds of cuts from the pro teams. Karl calls briefly daily, but he's somewhere out of my sphere right now, a place I can't even imagine. I am in limbo, suspended, waiting to see what's next in this life. But I'm comfortable and cocooned and safe while I wait.

Finally the call comes. "Janny! I made the team! I'm a Minnesota Viking! We're moving to Minneapolis, and this time we'll stay."

So once again I pack a U-Haul and make my way, alone, to Minneapolis, where Karl is already practicing with the team. The first regular season game is in one week, and Karl will be the starting strong safety—a position he will hold and start each game at for the next ten seasons.

When I arrive, we are over-the-top at both the good news and seeing each other again. It's been a long, anxious separation for newlyweds. After a few nights in a motel, we move into a new apartment complex in Bloomington. We furnish our small one-bedroom home with cheap, sticklike Danish modern furniture and the standard television-stereo console—it stores records on one side and has a television in the middle and a record player on the other side. Ours also has a built-in radio, so it is a little extra special.

Back at our Bloomington apartments, it's still warm, sunny September, and many other Vikings players are living in the same complex, so it's all very cozy. There are no roaches, and our clean one-bedroom apartment seems like the Hilton to me after all the sleaze of the past summer. We dump the black Ford for a new Dodge, light blue and cheap. And so ends a very strange but rich time, and I'm relieved to be settled. It's a good thing I have no idea of the steep learning curve I'll be required to complete in the next year.

+~+ +~+ +~+ +~+ +~+ +~+ +~+ +~+ +~+ +~+ +~+ +~+

Chapter 4

Rookie Wife

OW FOR THE BIG news: Karl has signed for a whopping nineteen thousand dollars for the season. Somehow I'd thought professional football players earned more, and I get a lesson in the hierarchies of the game. Both financially and socially, players operate on a tiered system. The highest paid are the offensive players, with the most going to the quarterbacks, then the premiere running backs, then the others on down. The salaries go down from there for the defense.

Rookies (first-year players at any position) are paid the least, unless they were Heisman Trophy winners or first-round draft picks. Of course, salaries go up with each year of play and are renegotiated each year. This is before there is a players' union, and the team manager could make a player feel as if each game lost was the player's fault, and thus cut the amount of raises. So salaries in general are not great, but that of a rookie defensive halfback is fairly small, though still about twice the national average for annual income at the time.

I will learn that no discussion or comparison of salaries is encouraged among the players. Like a group of codependents, the salary issue is kept secret, supposedly so as not to flare up rivalries. This big secret, though, actually only serves the owners, and I see that at once. But I'm never able to persuade any of the players that they need to band together, and if they do, they'll all be paid better. It will be many years before more powerful voices than mine develop the idea of players' representatives and a players' union.

Because of Karl's spending habits and his relatively low income, it quickly becomes apparent that our income will need to be supplemented. Although Karl gives me the money to manage, it soon becomes clear that he isn't giving me all of his income. He makes vague excuses and shrugs his shoulders, making it clear to me that I'll have to make do with this amount. I already realize a lot of money goes for beer. Much later in life, I will learn he was often fined for bad behavior and also loved to gamble.

So I need a job. Though I will not attend school at the University of Minnesota for the first quarter—it's too late to register and classes have already begun—I want to find employment there. These jobs are usually reserved for students. So I go over to the University of Minnesota and explain to the job office that I will be attending the university in the winter quarter, working on a bachelor of science degree. The job service personnel all recognize my name as the wife of the rookie defensive halfback who has already made a name for himself for speed and swift, solid tackling, as well as great runback skills in the preseason games. They find me a full-time job washing test tubes and glassware in a dental research lab, and off I go with my university career and contacts.

I go to work every day to stretch our funds, and Karl goes to practice every day with the Vikings. We buy two Siamese kittens, Plato and Mrs. Plato, to keep me company when Karl's gone (which will be often), and life swings into some relative normality.

The pregame routine is puzzling to me, but inflexible. If the game is at home, the men must spend the night before at the Thunderbird Motel near the football stadium in Bloomington, and they are not allowed any contact with their wives or families until after the game. Supposedly this is to avoid distracting them from the game with family issues or conflicts and to avoid expending energy on sexual relations with their wives (though I will learn soon enough that other women are fair game).

If the game is on the road, the team will fly out on a private plane on Thursday or Friday, have a practice or two on the other field on Saturday, and then play on Sunday (almost all games are on Sunday afternoons). On Sunday evening, all the players' wives line up at the arrival gate at the airport, along with fans, for the team's return.

The season begins, and Karl is starting. This is a good sign, but I quickly learn that there is no security of any kind in this job. Players are routinely cut throughout the season or traded to other teams. One injury, one missed game, or two or three bad errors could mean the end of your career at any time. Basically, players are meat to be bought, sold, traded, or discarded cynically and without feeling. It's just business. So the constant tension about staying on the team begins now.

It's a beautiful autumn day, and each Vikings player has two season tickets in the end zone under the shelter, just beneath the glassed-in reporters' box, in wide-open Metropolitan Stadium in Bloomington. I bring my friend Pat, a former sorority sister, who's married and thus not returning to Drake either, and we look around at the other Vikings wives. I don't know them yet, and many of them are old friends with each other, chatting away. They are sophisticated and well dressed. Some are stunning (I will learn that they are models). By their accents, I hear there are several Southern belles. No one introduces herself to me (I'm sure I look like some Iowa hick kid), so I decide to enjoy the game. Before long, Karl has made some great plays, and I find my shoulders being touched by Vikings wives who introduce themselves one by one. It seems they don't want to bother getting to know someone who will be there only a short time, as many rookie wives are, but it quickly becomes clear that Karl will likely become a fixture in the Vikings' secondary.

⊹◦⊹

THE VIKINGS team is just beginning to get going in the National League, led by quarterback Fran Tarkenton, famous for his scrambling, frantic play. Tarkenton is the son of a Georgia Methodist minister and neither drinks nor smokes—a rarity among the players. The quarterback and his wife are basically the pinnacle of the roster, both on and off the field.

The coach is a controversial rowdy named Norm Van Brocklin, who was probably very attracted to Karl's equally rowdy and rough-and-ready style of play. Norm can swear with the best of them, shout obscenities at the referees, and overturn barrels with his rage. He's a force of nature.

The team roster is made up of rejects and castoffs from other teams. Its first season ended with a last-place finish and a three-win, eleven-loss record. The second season had been even worse, with two wins, eleven losses, and one tie. I don't know it yet, but Karl and I will participate in some of the greatest years ever of the Vikings franchise, as the team improves each year. So the excitement at every game is huge, and the stadium is always sold out and packed. These are the salad years for this team, and we are part of it all.

This first home game is against the Chicago Bears, one of the prickly rivalries throughout Karl's playing years, and it is not a win for our team. But the Vikings had already defeated the San Francisco 49ers the previous week in California, so their record is now one win and one loss. The team goes on to finish the season with a more respectable five wins, eight losses, and one tie.

My understanding of football takes on new depths. I can really talk a good game now with anyone, including the players. And I begin to meet some serious Vikings fans, those who manage to give pregame parties in the parking lot for the players' and other fans, as well as those who succeed in getting the players to come to their homes or restaurants for parties after the games. I never understand how some maneuver themselves into this position, except for the obvious occasional sexy or rich woman. The celebrity life is on in full force here. Just rubbing shoulders with a player or his wife gives a person cache. So we are constantly surrounded by fans. Many of these people, who multiply daily, become my friends, although I will eventually learn the proper word is *acquaintances,* since they all immediately disappear from my life years later when Karl and I divorce.

After each game all the wives and the fans in the know wait at the end of a long tunnel for the guys to come out after their postgame lecture and shower. Only one guy refuses to shower after the game, and it becomes a popular joke among the waiting crowd, because he's always the first to come down the tunnel, and everyone can smell him coming from quite a distance. Maybe it's his clothes, or maybe he's been without a shower for more than a day. I don't know why he smells, except he doesn't shower after the game.

Depending on the outcome of the game, spirits will be high or low. It's not completely predictable, though, because if a player feels he didn't do well or made a mistake or was injured, winning does not lift his spirits. Depending on the player's spirits, the next stop may be a big party, a small party, a private party, a restaurant for dinner, or home. Some of the favorite restaurants over the years will be Shakey's Pizza, La Casa Coronada, The Embassy, or a country club. The player's wife never knows where or what the postgame event will be until after the game.

As the season goes on, the weather becomes very Minnesota-like. It is, as Karl would say, "Cold as a witch's tit in a brass bra!" Sitting there at five below zero and watching these games is a numbing experience. We all have to hold ourselves close for the little heat left, and we grit our teeth while smiling like beauty queens. It helps to have these strange half-sleeping bags, quilted and filled with goose down, that come up over the lower half of our bodies, but our dress must be in keeping with our celebrity, which usually means we are really freezing.

It's especially tough on the Southern women, but I suffer plenty too. My legs break out in gigantic hives when the weather is like this, and the itching is torture. We're always thrilled when halftime arrives, so we can rush to the rest room to warm up. But we must be in our seats when the game resumes. All eyes are on us, scrutinizing our behavior. Although we'd rather remain huddled together for warmth, we must jump up and cheer for every exciting play along with the rest of the crowd, no matter how we feel. And when we jump up, we lose all the reserve heat we've been working to store up.

A daily routine settles in. Karl has a playbook he studies, and the men have practice each day. Karl's good humor and funny laugh quickly earn him a place in the hearts of the team, while most rookies are usually on the outside for the first year. They all call him "Hunkie," and I never know for sure what that's about. Does it have to do with his build? Do they think he's Hungarian? Does it have something to do with his laugh? I don't know. I'm not even sure he knows, but it remains his affectionate nickname among the men for the rest of his career.

Karl's closest early friendships are quickly forged among other men of the defensive backfield: Dale Hackbart and Ed Sharockman, to name just a couple. And another daily routine develops over time. The boys take to drinking at the watering holes along I-494 before they come home after practice. At first, their drinking is within reason, but Karl occasionally comes home drunk, and sometimes he's very late, which means he has been driving drunk. His driving is as wild as his playing. And over the next nine years, he will be escorted home by the police from various venues at least twenty times. Drunk, driving, and speeding. He is never issued a ticket or even a warning.

⁌⊶⊷⁍

ONE VERY big advantage of football for Karl and me is his obvious ability to take out all his pent-up anger and aggressions on the field. So, with two exceptions, there is never violence in our marriage. This is a relief, given the modeling he's had in his upbringing. In fact, we rarely fight. We just have discussions of my concerns, which Karl generally laughs off.

We do have a fight over money early on in our new apartment, because his entire salary is paid out over three and a half months, and I have to make it stretch for the year. I can't see how it will stretch when Karl is pissing it away so quickly. Karl threatens with his fist, then slams it straight through the wall behind the front entry door, leaving a gaping six-inch hole.

Fortunately we have a wedding present we weren't planning on using. Now it has an immediate use. The plaque shows praying hands and has the inscription, "The family that prays together, stays together."

Behind a door is a bit of an odd place for a plaque to hang, but there it goes, and we'll eventually leave it there when we move on.

The season moves forward, and I'm surprised to receive an invitation to join the weekly bridge game with the elite among the Vikings wives. This invitation is unusual for either a defensive player's wife or a rookie's wife, so I understand it's an honor. I am grateful but not sure why I am chosen out in this way. I quickly learn bridge and love the gossip, camaraderie, and M&M's at each week's gathering. And I learn so very much about the culture of the Vikings, invaluable training that many other wives are not so fortunate to receive. I'll continue with the bridge group throughout my married years with Karl. Often some of us will get together to watch the away games on television.

Then one fine game day rolls around, and Karl is having his usual good game. He does make a few mistakes here and there throughout the year, but in general he is a very predictably good defensive halfback who plays his heart out for his team. He makes a vicious tackle and brings down an opposing halfback behind the line of scrimmage. The crowd goes wild.

But Karl doesn't get up. Here we go again. This time the television cameras swivel my way and also focus on the scene on the field. Karl seems to be unconscious. They are stimulating him, shouting at him, moving his limbs, taking off his helmet. Finally, he stirs and sits up. So he has a concussion, and I can see through my binoculars he has blood spurting from his nose. I assume he will sit out the next play, but he doesn't. He's right back on the field and continues his ferocious play. I'm not yet in medical school, but I know this can't be good for the brain—to go right back at whacks and bumps after an obvious concussion. But Karl correctly knows he has no choice. An injured player is of no use to the team, and he could easily lose his position by sitting out a play or two.

Over the next nine seasons, I'll see him with many concussions, a broken collarbone, a broken fibula, various sprains and ligamentous tears, and several broken noses. And this doesn't include the many injuries he had while playing college ball, including a fractured hand with plates and screws to knit it all together. He never misses a play. He will be on that field no matter what. Nobody at that time realizes what these beatings will do to their body in later life, and no one would listen anyway. These guys are in a love affair with their game. They are the lucky ones, the gods who are allowed to continue childhood pleasures into adulthood for money and celebrity. Playing is its own narcotic. No amount of pain or injury will keep them down. Of course, specialized taping and bracing from the team trainer helps a lot.

When Karl emerges from the tunnel after this game, his spirits are high, but his face isn't. He's not had any skin on the bridge of his nose for the entire preseason and regular season, as his helmet keeps hitting the prominence there. So I'm used to the white Band-Aid he constantly wears on his nose. But today this nose is obviously broken and smashed sideways. Apparently the team physician tried unsuccessfully to straighten it out, so Karl will just have to live with it until after the season, when a surgical repair will be in order. Until the surgery, he must breathe through his mouth, as his nose is completely blocked.

When he finally does have the surgery after the season is over, he is visited by a funny Irish Catholic priest in his room at St. Joseph's Hospital in St. Paul. I'm in the room when the priest comes breezing in, looking at the door name tag that says "Karl O. Kassulke."

The priest exclaims, "O'Kassulke! O'Kassulke! Sure and that's a funny Irish name!"

Even after my nineteenth birthday in November, I am still the youngest player's wife on the team. Because of my youth and the unlikely combination of the scholar-musician and football player, we have attracted the attention of the media as a couple, and some articles are even written about me alone. Of course there are many articles about Karl in the media on a regular basis.

Premiere sports columnist Jim Klobuchar interviews me one day at the university, and from the day that article is published in the *Star Tribune,* I have my own small celebrity as well as Karl's. Newspaper, magazine, radio, or television interviews become commonplace for both of us. Karl models for a national magazine article about pro football players. He wears a fur coat. The next season I buy him a marmot fur coat because of that article. He loves this coat, and it becomes his signature cold-weather wear for years. I will see photos of him in the media wearing that coat long after we are divorced.

I'm also carefully observing the groupies (attractive and horny women) who are everywhere we go. Generally, Karl doesn't pay much attention to them, at least when I'm around. But it's clear to me there are some dark sides to this celebrity stuff.

The other thing I notice increasingly is Karl's near obsession with celebrity, with being wanted and adored by his fans. He is not snotty— just the opposite. He will give the fans as much attention as they want, and he never charges for it, either (even when he goes out to speak to an organization). Other players are earning big extra money for their speaking engagements, but Karl receives nothing but the adulation he so very much needs. This is a rapidly growing monster that is spiraling quickly out of control.

One of the slivers that grows into a wedge between us is just this issue. As the years pass, Karl makes it plain that he can never be without this adulation. He begins immediately planning to own a restaurant and bar in order to keep the honey flowing. I am very against this because I already know that he will drink up all the profits while making merry with the customers. This begins as a small discussion during his first year of pro ball and grows into a mountainous argument by the time we part.

But in this first year the drinking and future needs are just whispers of trouble on the horizon. The major thing is that he's made it. He is great at what he does and will clearly have a career in pro ball. We both know this is a rare privilege, and both of us enjoy his well-earned celebrity and success. When one is eighteen or nineteen, what's not to enjoy about being a celebrity? Unfortunately, I have absolutely no understanding of the demands, sacrifices, and temptations rolling our way because of this celebrity.

The season ends with a happier coaching staff, and we prepare for the off-season. We don't really know what this will mean, either, but we shall soon find out.

Chapter 5

Summer Adventures

*A*FTER CHRISTMAS I START my sophomore year at the University of Minnesota. This is a campus of fifty thousand students, compared to Drake's two thousand. I've decided, for the time being, to major in medical technology. This course work is pure science, and I won't have another liberal arts class for the remainder of my college career. But I will play first-chair cello in the university orchestra during my undergraduate years. At this time, this is not an outstanding orchestra. And I'll also sing in a very accomplished church choir at Richfield Methodist Church, which puts on a big spectacle each Easter and otherwise is a well-honed musical group, nearly as professional as I'm used to. And I find another orchestra to play in, the Bloomington Symphony, which is conducted by famous jazz musician Paul Wesley "Doc" Evans. So it's unique and also semiprofessional. These activities fill my musical needs for the time being.

Medical technology is designed to prepare graduates to run the laboratories at hospitals or do research. It's a four-and-a-half-year program. I've already finished one, and I've chosen it as an alternative to premed because of great disapproval and pressure from Karl's parents regarding medical school. But I've already discovered that most of the course work is identical to premed, and some is in even greater depth. Many of the upper division classes are actually attended by both medical technologists and medical students.

I find I'm one of two new persons in the already tightly bonded forty-person subgroup of medical technology majors, so I am on the outside for a bit until I get to know everyone. The other new student is Susan from Edina, who also has transferred in. She is cute, petite, blond, and well dressed, and we sit together in all our classes. We have fun in one class, microbiology, because there is a male premed student with a reputation for womanizing who is dying to sit next to Susan. She always engineers things so that someone sits on one side of her, and I sit on the other, so this guy can't get what he wants. After weeks of frustration, he stops me when we are walking up the aisle at the end of class.

"You big horse! Why don't you get out of the way and let me sit next to Susan?"

I don't even answer him because I'm so shocked. Big horse? Shades of high school all over again! Now I'm at least mature enough to understand his motives for saying such a thing, but still it hurts. I vow to show him, as is often the motivation for my overachieving. And sure enough, at medical school graduation, I will show him.

All together this university experience is very different than Drake. America is entering a time of dramatically liberalized ideas for women and students, and I wear jeans and shorts to classes. The classes have several hundred students in each, and the professors and teaching assistants don't pay any attention to who attends and who doesn't. The main thing is what the student accomplishes on the tests. Otherwise, we're mostly anonymous. Many of us are fairly casual about attendance. If we miss a day or two here and there, we just get the notes from one of our friends, and that takes care of it. Of course, I'm the only married student in this group, so I miss more classes than most. Married life does have some extra demands.

Before long, though, I'm no longer anonymous on this huge campus. I'm the wife of sports celebrity Karl Kassulke, and nearly everyone speaks to me or smiles, and professors know who I am. Now I'm under a microscope. Most folks obviously wish me well and cheer me on, but I'm aware of some jealousies and hopes that I will fail. There definitely are pressures I haven't experienced before.

I've missed the first quarter of my sophomore year, so I am now behind in some classes. I'll need to attend summer school every year in order to graduate. In the end, it will take me five years to finish the medical technology program.

⌘

THE PROSPECT of so much more school ahead doesn't bother me especially, as I like learning and exploring. I don't like mathematics, however, and choose not to take any advanced math, like calculus. I've already fulfilled the basic mathematics requirements, and that's plenty for me. Before I graduate, I will have completed in-depth chemistry, microbiology, biology, psychology, biochemistry, anatomy, and physics, as well as laboratory science and electronics (in order to know how to maintain the rapidly evolving technology that will autoanalyze blood).

What does concern me is money. The football season is over, and we have very little reserve. School is not expensive—about $150 a quarter—so that isn't an issue. But we still have only one car, and my lab job is just squeaking us by.

Then, through my immunology professor, I meet a researcher, Dr. Edmond Yunis, who gives me a job as a research assistant in his lab. This lab is exploring the early new ideas about antigens and antibodies—immunology—as they relate to the new science of kidney transplantation and cancer. My pay in this lab is up one notch on the university pay scale, so that helps a bit. I love the challenge and the creative detective work of this world, and I'll work in the same lab between twenty and forty hours a week the rest of the time I am in undergraduate and medical school.

Meanwhile, I notice many of the Vikings players have off-season jobs, aided in their placement by Vikings supporters. Many seem to be earning well, and the opportunities for speaking engagements and appearances are plentiful, also a source of money. But Karl is very casual about these things. He wants to please everyone. He's flattered at the speaking opportunities and doesn't press for any pay. As a result, no pay is offered, and he rapidly gets the reputation of speaking for free. Very quickly these free speaking commitments keep him away from home many nights every week. These events fill his need for adulation, but that well never stays full for long. I can't seem to get him to stand up for himself and request the money due him. His need to please his fans gets in the way of our needs as a family again and again. It's truly frustrating for me, as I just look around and see all the activities of the other Vikings players and see such a different picture with us when it comes to earning money.

Then Karl takes a job as an insurance salesman. One of those super Vikings fans has managed to get close enough to him and offered him this job, which will not pay unless he sells policies. Soon I discover Karl is actually paying the people to buy the insurance, because he feels sorry for them if they can't afford it. So once again, he has no money coming in for his efforts. Instead, it goes out at jet speed.

Another off-season friendship that Karl develops is with a fellow who owns a large and successful business in downtown Minneapolis. We are his guests there frequently, and we meet his wife, who is a star at the Guthrie Theater. I see very quickly that this man, "R," is bisexual and is sexually fixated on Karl. Karl, however, is oblivious to all the flatteries, the attempts to sit extra close, the special meals at his business, and the constant invitations to galas and in-crowd events. This first year R confines himself to staying as close to Karl as he can, while at the same time he's obviously buttering me up so I will not stop the relationship.

"Jan, you know I love Karl. I have to have him. I won't break up your relationship."

"R, is that why you sent me two dozen roses?"

"Well, you're my friend too, and there's no reason we can't be adult about this."

"What does that mean—being adult?"

"Well, these are open times. My wife knows about this, and she accepts it. So maybe you can too."

"R, I don't have any problem being friends with you two. You're fun to be with. But I certainly do have a problem with Karl having a sexual relationship with anyone else—man or woman. Besides, Karl may not say no very clearly, but believe me, when it comes to you, he will mean no."

"Well, we'll see about that. I can be pretty persuasive."

"I'm sure you can, and Karl can be very pliable. But I know him well enough to know he'll be repulsed if you make a move on him. It would probably backfire on you, and you'd lose him as a friend."

"I just can't give up hope. I dream about him night and day."

"R, you're going to have a breakdown if you don't get a grip. Karl just isn't for you, and that's that."

I tell Karl what's going on, in detail, but he doesn't worry. And R's wife is fine. I enjoy her company. But this couple's relationship with us will eventually and inevitably develop into a very dark chapter.

The off-season passes in this way. Karl and the guys occasionally work out or see the team trainer. They go out drinking a lot at night. Karl is often gone speaking or appearing somewhere. I cook great meals for him, and he loves to eat at home. We play lots of cribbage and cuddle with each other and our cats.

I work five days a week, and we socialize with our friends, who are all either players or fans, plus my friend from Drake, Pat Billbe Lindquist, her new husband, and their new baby girl, who will become our godchild. I go to school daily and carry more than a full load of classes in order to catch up. Gradually I'm accepted into the tightly knit group of med tech students. I'm home alone many nights, so there's always time to get schoolwork done.

Then, over a school break, we go to Las Vegas on an NFL-sponsored trip. We meet many players and their wives from other teams, and it's fun to see them in person instead of as opponents on the field. The trip is great for us because we only need to pay airfare. Everything else is free, including meals and shows. Basically we are human advertising for the Sands Casino and Hotel.

We're treated royally for free and booked into a luxury suite. My, what a long way we've come in less than a year! We enjoy private seats in the front booths for each show, but I am totally shocked at the nudity! We go backstage and joke with Liberace, a famous flamingly gay piano player who, it turns out, is from Milwaukee. So he adores Karl. (He probably would have adored him if he were from Timbuktu!) They talk, reminiscing about the good old days in Milwaukee, and laugh long. Liberace gives me two signed record albums and shows me his collection of outrageous, gaudy rings. Every finger on his hands sports one of his hundreds of jeweled rings. In his dressing room, Liberace wears a pink-fur-and-feathers dressing gown as we chat.

We're shepherded everywhere in the Sands by the entertainment director, a sleazy man in a pink jacket with a constantly chewed cigar in his mouth. He's tall, bulky, sweaty, crude, and overbearing. He invades my personal space constantly with his stinking cigar breath, and I have to endure him in order to get all the goodies we're promised.

We meet all the Las Vegas show biz celebrities: Frank Sinatra, Ed McMahon (I will meet him again in New Orleans), Sammy Davis Jr., Tony Bennett, and Dean Martin. They are all polite and chat for a moment, but it's clear they've already had their fill of meeting and greeting, football players or not. I can see they'd like their own lives to live, and I don't want to spend time with them, sensing their restless boredom. I contemplate this and see my future.

Nevertheless, I love Las Vegas. It's exotic, way beyond anything I could imagine (though by 2010 it's completely over the top). I discover I can play blackjack all day and never lose any money. I earn about ten dollars for the day. I am very cautious with my bets and never double down or take any risks that would mean losing money faster. Most of the dealers use one or two decks, and one-dollar bets are the standard, so it's very easy to count cards and keep track of the best move to make on any given hand. And all the soft drinks are free! It's just too much! Karl occupies himself elsewhere. Usually I don't know what he's up to, besides drinking, but we always meet somewhere at the correct time.

One day I'm alone downtown, playing nickel slot machines, when a strange older woman comes over to me. I can remember the low-cut blue miniskirt dress with yellow dots I wore (times are changing very fast regarding clothing). She says, "You're very young and beautiful, and I want to help you. Let me show you."

I don't know what to make of this, but she seems harmless. She takes me to a different slot machine and instructs me to play just this machine and none other. After ten minutes, I startle and scream when I win a ten-dollar jackpot. She says, "No, wait, don't stop now. Keep playing the same machine."

Reluctantly, I do as she says, and suddenly, when it looks like my ten dollars will be gone, I hit a one-hundred-dollar jackpot. Everyone goes crazy and comes over at the loud bells and clanging coins. She waits until I collect my money, then takes me aside and says, "Now the smart gambler will take her money and stop for the day. Do you understand?"

I do, and I quit. I have about two hundred dollars more when we return home than when I came to Las Vegas. It's great!

ᐟᑌᐠ

THE SCHOOL year is grinding to the end of the third quarter, and money, as usual, is tight. But it's time for Karl to have his first private meeting with Jim Finks, the general manager of the Vikings, to renegotiate his contract. Karl's had a good year and proved his value to the team, and I have high hopes. But when Karl comes home, he's looking at the floor as he tells me his negotiated salary for next season. He will receive a two-thousand-dollar raise. I can't understand why so little. I know many Vikings receive much larger salaries. Then Karl begins to describe the scene.

He met with Finks in the film room at the training facility. Finks had put together film of Karl's every missed tackle, every fluffed fumble recovery, every short runback. Not one image of his good or great plays of the last season.

In this way Karl is demoralized and is hoping to keep his position. He thinks that he must be such a lousy player. At this point, Finks pats him on the back and says, "Well, we'll give you another chance this year. I don't think you've earned more than a two-thousand-dollar raise. Do you?"

Karl quickly agrees. He is happy to keep his position. This is how each negotiation will go every year, with about a raise of two thousand dollars per year, even when Karl is an all pro. Excluding bonuses for postseason games, the most he ever earns in any one season is around thirty-two thousand dollars.

With his contract signed and a few days off before I start summer school, we travel down to Boone for a few days with my family. I have time to show him some of my favorite haunts, like the beautiful Ledges State Park. We run barefoot through the cold streams that course over the roadbeds and receive the usual dousing when kids in cars see us and speed through the streams to splash us. Pizza is still fairly new, but Boone has the Tic Toc Lounge, where a spicy thin-crust pizza—my favorite—is ordered by phone and must be picked up through a back-alley window since I'm not of drinking age in Iowa.

We both relax while my mom pampers us with her great cooking, and I try to keep the celebrity stuff to a minimum. Of course, this means we don't see many old friends, though I'm discovering we now have very little in common anyway. High school friends really are by-gone friends for now. I've moved on to a world of marriage and celebrity. I never imagined this would be so. But it is, and that's that.

Our best adventure in Boone this trip is a surprise collision with a black angus bull. Karl and I are driving in the countryside one night, and then the road is suddenly blocked by a gigantic black bull that scrambles out of a ditch right into the front of our car. Although we brake, there's no way to avoid hitting this behemoth.

The bull is knocked flat, and our lights are all smashed out. It's a very dark night, so we can't exactly see what happened to the bull. Cautiously, we get out of our little blue Dodge and look for the bull. We find him by the sound of his snorting. He's struggling to get to his feet. When he manages to get up, we can see the white part of his eyes when he looks at us. I guess he decides one smack from a car is enough, so he abruptly turns, jumps the ditch, and trots off into the field.

It's my first car accident, and I have no idea what to do next. Should we try to find the farmer and tell him about his bull? How can we get home with no lights (not even a flashlight)? Will our car even work?

Fortunately, the car starts right up, and we inch along in the moon-less night until we finally reach the streetlight safety of Boone. Once home, a car inspection reveals we now have a big front-end scrunch on our Dodge. We never do get it fixed, due to the insurance deductible. It drives fine, so why bother?

Back in Minneapolis, I start the first of two summer quarters, catching up on some advanced chemistry and biology classes I missed the previous year. Karl and the rest of the guys relax. In a few brief days, they'll be gone again to Bemidji for training camp, and I'll be alone again well into September. When he leaves, Karl doesn't give me any funds, so I'll need to survive on my work salary. I've received a raise already, so that helps.

But round two is about to start. It seems likely Karl will make the team, but no one is assured of that until after the last cuts in September. And this team, like most, has drafted one or more rookies who play Karl's position, so the competition and anxiety never lets up.

Chapter 6

Alone Again, Naturally

*A*UGUST 1964: Karl and the team depart for training camp. Karl rides to camp with a buddy, so at least I have a car. I've finished summer school for this year, but I still go to work daily. Karl will receive $150 a week this year during training camp, but none of it comes to me. I'm getting by on my salary but have no extra money.

Karl doesn't call every day this year. We're both less anxious about his future, but there is still the constant worry about injury. Also, Karl has to fight to keep his spot because of those newly drafted defensive backs. But this time he's the experienced player, and each training camp will be the same from now on. New defensive backs come in to try for his job, but they're never successful.

And we aren't newlyweds anymore. The "oh, wow" period is over, and we're both more mature, though we've already begun to grow in different directions. I'm getting job experience, making connections at the University of Minnesota, and stretching my brain with truly tough courses. At the same time, Karl is expanding his fan base, learning new ways to charm people, figuring out how to stay on the team by improving his game and his knowledge of his opponents, and growing more rowdy and reckless with his off-field behavior.

I have no idea how to halt this steady slide into reckless driving and drinking. No one seems to want to get involved, so I'm on my own. The rest of his best buddies on the team are doing the same thing. Not all players deteriorate in this direction, just Karl's circle of rowdy, heavy-drinking risk takers. It seems like that wild thing that inhabits their very core and makes them such stellar football players is also what they increasingly bring to their lives off the field, and my concern is steadily growing. This is a long time before anyone we know understands or cares about Alcoholics Anonymous (though it does exist), codependency, or all the other problems and solutions associated with heavy alcohol use. I certainly have no knowledge or experience to bring to this issue of problematic alcohol behavior.

One of my priorities during this time apart from Karl is to figure out why I haven't gotten pregnant. We've never used birth control, and Karl is getting restless. Most of the other Vikings have families already, and despite my youth, he wants to get started. So I visit the Viking wives' obstetrician, a doctor who will eventually become my friend and admirer. Later, when he's president of the exclusive Edina Rotary Club, he'll bring me along to a meeting as his guest at a time when women are not allowed at Rotary meetings.

For now, William Stromme, a doctor so prominent that the obstetrics wing at Abbott Northwestern Hospital will eventually be named for him, becomes my doctor. He is very busy, kind, attentive, and grandfatherly, and always available to me for any reason. Even when he's not on call, he'll be certain to be available for my needs, though this is certainly not the norm for obstetricians.

When he completes my exam, he tells me I have endometriosis, which can make it difficult to conceive, plus another minor problem that he can fix with a small office procedure. He doesn't explain the procedure, but I'm intrigued when smoke and the smell of burning flesh rises from behind the modesty sheet. There's some cramping associated with this, and I don't enjoy it. When the procedure is over, Dr. Stromme warns me to avoid sexual relations for two weeks—not a problem since Karl is gone. "After Karl returns," he says, "you'll be pregnant in no time. You'll see. Don't worry about that endometriosis."

Pregnancy and having children is not anything I question at this point in my life. Society expects every wife to start a family, so it seems perfectly reasonable to me at all of age nineteen to bring little lives into my circle. I expect to love them and cherish them, and I can't wait to see their sweet faces. I know absolutely nothing about parenting, but then, who does?

✦

THE LATE summer days drag on. Though I am playing weekly bridge, I do very little other socializing. Mainly my cats keep me company at home. One small drama occurs when Plato, a tomcat, jumps off the second-floor balcony, apparently in search of some variety from Mrs. Plato. It takes me an anxious half day to find him mewing dejectedly under a building overhang three buildings away. No more balcony visits for this guy!

Plato provided a different sort of excitement the previous Thanksgiving. He is not neutered, and this is my first experience of an entirely indoor cat. He has been teaching me about the delights of a male cat spraying to mark his territory.

This particular Thanksgiving I have made my signature pumpkin chiffon cake from scratch. Everyone raves about it being better than pumpkin pie. Karl isn't home. The Vikings play an away game on Thanksgiving Day every year, so he always misses both Thanksgiving and my birthday, which often falls on Thanksgiving Day. So my parents have come to visit for the holiday. After a full-on traditional Thanksgiving feast, I proudly bring the cake down from its perch on the top of the refrigerator. I slather whipped cream on each slice, and we all dig in. I notice it first, then both my parents politely put down their forks.

My beloved stinker cat has sprayed this cake. It had never dawned on me that he would get on top of the refrigerator, risking a tangle with the pilot light on the stove top. He has already burned his tail once on this pilot light. But jump on the refrigerator he does, and he sprays this particular cake just this time. It really is an indescribably nasty taste!

We all laugh it off, toss the beautiful cake out, and settle for the other dessert: pumpkin pie.

Cats will prove to be my trusty, reliable companions throughout my adult years, though they can be rascals. Through great times, kitten times, baby times, difficult times, human failings and abandonments, and tragedies, my cats will always, without fail, respond to my moods and share fun or healing with me. I guess this is what pets are all about.

Besides cats, I have a love of all nature and am fascinated with the preservation of wildlife. Because of this, I get into quite a bind this particular preseason. I've been coming home each day from work at the university via a route that takes me over the Mississippi River at the

---

PUMPKIN CHIFFON CAKE

Here's my recipe for pumpkin chiffon cake. I recommend you leave out the cat spray.

2 cups sifted all-purpose flour
1½ cups sugar
3 teaspoons baking powder
1 teaspoon salt
1 teaspoon ground cinnamon
½ teaspoon each ground cloves and grated nutmeg
½ cup canola oil
8 egg yolks
½ cup water
¾ cup pumpkin
½ teaspoon cream of tartar
8 egg whites

In a large bowl, sift the dry ingredients together. Make a well in the center. Add, in order, the oil, egg yolks, water, and pumpkin. Beat until satin smooth. In another large bowl, add the cream of tartar to the egg whites and beat to very stiff peaks. Pour the yolk batter in a thin stream over the entire surface of the whites, gently folding in to blend. Bake in an ungreased 10-inch tube pan at 325° for 55 minutes. Increase the heat to 350° and bake another 10 minutes. Invert the pan to cool. Remove the cake when cool and serve with sweetened whipped cream.

Washington Avenue Bridge, then along Minnehaha Parkway and around Lake Nokomis. There are no through freeways as yet, and Cedar Avenue is the fastest route. As I cross the Washington Avenue Bridge this day, the unexpected happens.

A very large snapping turtle—probably twenty-four inches in diameter—is in the middle of the road. He will surely be squashed, as traffic is brisk. Without a thought, I stop my car and pick up this stinking, struggling, threatening, hissing, prehistoric-looking snapper and put him in my trunk. I'll drop him in Lake Nokomis when I pass by.

When I reach Lake Nokomis, I park not ten feet from the water. I take the keys out of the ignition, then realize I can't hold them and the turtle both without getting hurt. So, since I'm so close to the lake, I drop the keys into my purse on the front seat, then take the struggling turtle to the lake, where he quickly swims away without a backward glance.

I'm back at my car within two minutes, but my purse is gone, as are the keys! I'm stunned and starkly dejected. How could this happen? I tell myself no good deed goes unpunished. I'll learn this again and again as I age.

Now what? I've lost forty dollars, which is all the money I have, and it had to last for a week. I don't have the keys to start the car, and all my identification and credit cards are gone, along with precious pictures of my loved ones, including Karl.

I'm overwhelmed, and I sit on the front of the car and bawl and sob. I have no idea what to do. I can't even get into my apartment. I can't lock my car because I don't know how I'd get it open again. This is all new for me, before I've learned about locksmiths and police hooks that quickly unlock cars. I don't know what to do.

A passing motorist sees me sobbing on the front hood of my car and stops to help. When I give him my name, he snaps to and says he'll do anything I need. How can he help?

He says, "We'll lock up the car, then take you to your apartment in Bloomington. Then we'll find your apartment manager. He can let you into your apartment. I'll bet you have an extra set of keys, yes?"

"I do," I reply, because Karl's keys are hanging on a nail beside the praying hands plaque. So off we go, this indignant Vikings fan driving

me home and smoothing my way. When we find the apartment manager, he's fuming that someone should do this to a Vikings wife, and he
swings into outraged action.

Once I have my extra set of keys, the apartment manager takes me
back to Lake Nokomis, but instead of going directly to my car, he begins to drive around the lake.

"What are you doing?" I ask. "My car's over there on the other side
of the lake."

"I'm going to find the bastard who stole your stuff and teach him a
good lesson!"

I have no idea how he plans to find the culprit, so I just slump in
the seat and think about how I will get some temporary money. Suddenly, there he is. A teenager is sneaking along the street side of cars
whose owners are on the lake side and can't see his hunched-over
body. He peeks into each car, and we actually see him reach in and grab
a camera from an open window. That does it.

The burly apartment manager slams on the brakes and jumps out
of the car, grabs the kid by the scruff of his neck, and starts slamming
him repeatedly into a car. The air is blue with his swearing, echoing out
over the lake and the many frolicking people. Finally I step in because
I'm afraid he'll seriously hurt the kid. I say, "Let's take him to the small
police station just on the other side of the lake."

So the thoroughly scared teenager is thrown into the front seat with
his neck in a vise grip from the manager's big hand, and we travel the
short distance to the police station. There he repeatedly denies stealing
my purse, though he can hardly deny stealing the camera since he has it
in his backpack, and we both witnessed his thievery. Finally, he admits
to stealing the purse and agrees to lead us to it. Two policemen, the
apartment manager, and I troop to a nearby trash bin. The ashen-faced
boy reaches inside and pulls out a purse. Unfortunately, it isn't mine.

So someone gets her purse back, and a little thief gets caught, but
I'm left without my stuff. It will keep me busy getting a new license,
credit cards, and photos. The apartment manager loans me some
money for a few weeks, and I'm back in business. I sure hope that
damn turtle is happy!

Four years later I get a phone call from a woman who identifies herself as living near Lake Nokomis. She asks me if I had a purse stolen. I have to think a moment because it's been so long. When I remember, I say, "That was four years ago. Why are you asking now?"

"Well," she says, "my little boy was digging in the sand today at the lake, and there was your purse with all your identification and license still there. No money or credit cards, though."

So after all those years, I get everything back except the money and credit cards. Even the pictures have been preserved inside the good quality leather of the purse.

Lake Nokomis is a place Karl and I frequent in the summers when we live in Bloomington, beginning with our first summer there. We have figured out that we can catch some fish off the Cedar Avenue Bridge, with traffic whizzing by, and I discover I'm talented at fishing. I seem to know just when to surprise set a hook, though I have not grown up knowing how to fish. Iowa is not known for its lakes, and the river fish are bullheads or muddy catfish. My mother's preparation of these fish, brought home by my brothers, turns me off all seafood and items from water forever. I can't get the memory of that muddy taste and texture out of my mind.

But I like to fish, just as long as someone else cleans and eats them. It's not uncommon for me to hook a fish in the side instead of in the mouth, just because I felt the fish brushing the line. Then I have to haul it up the fifteen feet or so from the lake on to the bridge. My best catches off this bridge are big northern pikes, sunfish, and some pretty good bass too.

So I go fishing alone occasionally on my way home from work while Karl is in training camp (carefully locking my car after my lesson in theft). I keep some worms and a bucket in the car, along with a cheap fishing pole. It's tricky not to lose the wiggling fish in the long haul up from the river, but I master it well. Though I don't eat fish, it's fine for the cats and for stocking the freezer for Karl's return.

Finally, the long training camp is over, and Karl returns happy and laughing. He's successfully beat out the rookies, kept his position, and had a good run so far in the preseason games.

Of course, first things first, and we head immediately for the sack when we get home from the airport. As it happens, I conceive on Karl's very first day home from training camp. It will be a few weeks before I know this, but very soon everything changes.

Chapter 7

Dark Clouds Forming

SEPTEMBER 1964: With the coming of clear, fine, blue-sky autumn days free of the summer misery of ticks and mosquitoes, a new season opens for the Vikings. I'm beginning to see how the cycle of my life will circle for the next many years. It revolves around football, starting with the football season, with celebrity, and with anxiety and worry over performance and injuries—all at a fever pitch. Then comes the next off-season and money worries and the escalation each year of wild behavior and unpredictable changes in Karl. Then he is gone again for training camp, and round and round it will go. The other constants during all that will be my steady job, my studies at the University of Minnesota, my cats, and, soon enough, my kids.

Nineteen sixty-four is season number four for the Minnesota Vikings and season two for Karl Kassulke. The team has added some important depth at some positions, especially Carl Eller as the first seed of what will eventually be known as the Purple People Eaters, a fearsome foursome of defensive linemen. But on both the offense and defense some players have been replaced by stronger and better players, and other players are gelling and maturing. All predictions are for a stronger finish this year, so hopes are high for a better season.

The fans are crazy about their team, especially when they're winning. The St. Paul–Minneapolis area is a relatively small market for a major league football team, and everyone is grateful and proud to have not only professional football but also hockey and baseball franchises. The operative impact here for the players is "relatively small," for they are told they are playing in the smallest stadium and thus have the lowest salaries, making it difficult to attract star players. In later years I will look up the statistics and learn this is a myth. The Vikings and the Twins, who both used the Metropolitan Stadium, were very profitable—for the owners.

But these guys have to make it against much bigger teams (like Los Angeles and New York) and markets—and they do. They are all heart and devil-may-care on the field, and it works. They all play as if there is no tomorrow. Even I do not yet fully realize the toll this will take on every aspect of their lives.

So the routine starts up again: Karl gone the night before the game or flying out on the Friday before an away game. My parents come up from Boone for at least one game each season, and Karl's parents also come in from Milwaukee at least once each fall. These visits from Karl's parents are tense, though Otto's behavior is better than when he is on his home turf. They are so very proud of their boy and rightfully so. Hopefully that blunts some of Otto's disappointment and anger with his own life.

The players' wives trade tickets back and forth so we can take two others with us to games when we have guests. Our seats are in the same place in the stadium for all of Karl's playing days, so the wives become a close-knit group while sitting through the joys, disappointments, injuries, thrills, freezing cold, and pride of each game while our spouses do what they do best.

For one game I've brought along an old friend from Boone: Tim Croxen. The fans are especially excited this day, as it's a close game. Eventually the Vikings lose. On the way down the spiral ramp that leads from our seats on the upper deck, a group of drunken fans becomes very rowdy and threatening, right next to me. They shout lewd suggestions at me. They have no idea who I am.

"Hey, sweetie, want a bite of my hot dog?"

"Listen, darlin', I've got some good sausage for you. Just come with me to my car," and then he grabs my arm and tries to drag me.

Tim tells them to pipe down. They respond by picking him up by his feet and holding him over the edge of the safety bars on the ramp.

"Think you're a hero, huh?"

"Think you can handle a hottie like this? We'll take care of her!"

It's a terrifying moment. It looks like they're going to drop Tim on his head onto the concrete floor three stories below, and they're really drunk and unpredictable. I'm screaming for help, but there is only milling chaos as everyone rushes to get out of the stadium and into some warmth somewhere. I'm not even sure anyone sees what's going on.

Finally a group of strong men intervenes, and after a few well-placed punches to the outside of the pack, they reach Tim's legs and pull him to safety. Tim is nearly unconscious from hanging upside down, and he is ghostly pale. There is more shouting and confusion. No policemen intervene, because the drunkards scatter before any law enforcement can arrive. It's another scary lesson for me in how quickly circumstances can turn deadly when alcohol is involved.

My pregnancy doesn't show yet. Ultrasound has not yet been invented, so I don't know if I'm carrying a boy or a girl. Everyone knows I'm pregnant, though, as both Karl and I have joyously announced it. Our baby will be due about the second week in June 1965. I'm thinking, "How convenient. I can finish the entire school year before the birth." But I've developed quite serious vomiting already, and I'm enormously sleepy, snoozing as much as twenty hours a day some days. I'm vomiting from morning to night and can't find any food to stay down, except for red licorice.

The vomiting is a problem for the postgame gatherings. I avoid eating so as not to upchuck too often during these events when all eyes are on the Vikings and their wives. One night, though, we all gather at a Shakey's Pizza on I-494, not far from the stadium and not far from an apartment complex where many Vikings players live. I love pizza. I think it's God's food, along with bacon and cheese, so I indulge and eat some delicious pizza. Bad idea.

Suddenly, I run for the bathroom and vomit forcefully into the toilet, the chunks of undigested pizza splashing out of the toilet and onto my face and clothes. I am so repulsed by this that it will be years before I can eat pizza again or go to Shakey's.

✦

THE BIGGEST rivalry for the Vikings is the Green Bay Packers. They are an older and much stronger team, and they consistently win the division title. They are packed with stars. Their quarterback is even named Bart *Starr.* And their fans are rabid. This year I will attend my first away game and take my first flight, which in retrospect is not a good decision given my vomiting problems. But I get on the short flight that will bounce down twice at small airports before landing at Green Bay. I quickly become a veteran of the barf bag. It's a very turbulent ride, and every bump of the relatively small plane makes me vomit anew, as does every takeoff and landing. It's a completely miserable flight, and I have very little chance to enjoy any sights from the air. The stewardesses are obviously uncomfortable with my level of sickness and hover over me, their brows furrowed. There's nothing to be done but get through it.

The Green Bay game at Lambeau Field is a surprising win at the last minute for the Vikings (24–23), so there's much jubilation among the small Vikings contingent at the game. Karl's parents are there as well, because Green Bay is not far from Milwaukee. So we all (the fans and Karl's family) have a restaurant stop before I get to the airport for the flight home.

Once I am on the plane, I do a repeat barfing performance. So far, I'm not very excited about flying, but the future will prove that the vomiting was only because of my pregnancy. In my lifetime I will travel well over a million miles in the air and never again have a vomiting problem.

Back at the Metropolitan Stadium, a peculiar incident takes place in the women's rest room during a game halftime. Elaine Tarkenton, the quarterback's wife, approaches me while I'm washing my hands.

We're all hanging around in the rest room to warm up, and Elaine is a friend by now, as we play bridge together each week. But she says to me in her Georgia accent, "You know, y'all are the most improved Viking wife this season."

She doesn't elaborate, and I don't know what to make of this. Is it a complement? Does it mean I was a slug or a slob last year? I just don't know and don't have the quick wits to ask her what she means. I just thank her and go on with washing my hands, but suddenly I wonder if my every move is being judged by a group of women who consider themselves my superior and are now awarding me in a way for changing somehow to be more like them.

And there is a subtle change occurring among many of the men, including Karl, after the game. They seem to be high on adrenalin and need more alcohol to bring themselves down. Some are talking faster than usual, and some even have jitters or can't sit still, or they laugh more often and louder than usual. There's a strange disquiet developing that I don't understand. It never turns violent, but it's an uncomfortable feeling. And I watch the men drink more and more alcohol, usually beer.

Finally I ask Karl about this change. He just shrugs and says, with his usual laugh, which accompanies nearly every thing he has to say, "They give us this pill in the locker room to help our game, and it makes us tense and jittery. I think I play better when I take it." He doesn't know what the pill is, but he says, "After the game, some guys take another pill to help them relax, but most of us just do it with beer."

This is all he'll say on this subject this season. He never says who "they" are, and I don't ask. I have no idea if this is a sanctioned Viking activity or if there is a pill pusher in the locker room operating beneath the radar. We will return to this discussion each season, however, and each time there will be additional changes in the drugs used before and after the games.

One day after practice, the guys are on their usual rounds of bars before coming home, when I get a call that Karl is too drunk to drive. Can I come and pick him up? This is a rarity, as the wives are never included in these drinking rounds, and we're not even allowed to know where the guys are at any particular time. When I arrive at the restaurant-bar on I-494, Karl is passed out on a table. The rest of the guys have pitchers of beer on their tables and are surrounded by pretty women, none of whom are their wives, but all of whom are obviously hoping to become wives. They are physically hanging onto the shoulders and arms of the guys, who are all married, of course. A few are kissing or pushing their breasts into drunken faces.

So this is the drinking scene. I am pregnant and miserable, and Karl and the guys are partying with other women. I see that I just better get used to it and hope he can stay faithful, but my heart actually sinks. I don't know if he can resist these women forever, because he is so easygoing and so quick to say yes to whatever is going on. I know that marriages mature, and children and other responsibilities develop, thus other women will seem more exciting. With all the beer and drugs involved, I hope against hope that Karl can be true to his family.

School during this football season is back on track because my summer school classes have completely caught me up, and now I'm synchronized with the rigid schedule of the medical technology curriculum. This junior year at university is a cycle of classes that are only done once a year and in specific quarters. So I must go to school every quarter or fall a year behind, pregnancy sickness or not.

I find myself getting up early, driving to the university, then squeezing behind a couch in Coffman Union and sleeping on the floor. I miss a lot of classes, but I'm able to get notes from my classmates to keep myself caught up. One class, in particular—hematology—which I dearly love, proves to be the biggest challenge. The class involves microscopic examinations for the entire hour. Every movement of the slide under the scope makes me nauseous, and I run to vomit many times during each class. Somehow, though, I get through the quarter with decent grades, but it's really no fun.

I'm planning ahead this year, so one day I take Karl with me to a home development site I've scouted out in Burnsville, just across the Minnesota River from Bloomington. There are five model homes on a large tract of bare land in this suburb of 5,000 people—eventually it will be 110,000. I've decided I want a home here, and I want it to be ready when the baby comes. I also see this home purchase as a way to get some of Karl's income put away before it's pissed away.

I've already decided on a contemporary three-bedroom, split-level home, about twenty-four hundred square feet, and Karl is eager to go along with this big purchase. We easily get a mortgage for this twenty-two-thousand-dollar home, make the down payment while we still have a chunk of money, and make our choices for lighting, paint, flooring, cabinets, and décor. We're committed to our first real house. Its completion date is May 1, so my plans are to move in right before our family expands.

When I'm just three months pregnant and before I really show yet, the expanding baby reveals for us a weakness of my abdominal skin. The skin begins to split, with ugly red, bleeding, half-inch-wide vertical stretch marks covering my abdomen up to my rib cage. Karl is horrified. At first he seems sympathetic, but very soon he cannot either look at me or touch me. Though he will still make love to me, it is always with his face averted from what he obviously considers a terrible disfigurement on my belly. He will never touch my abdomen again— not to feel the baby move, not to try to hear the baby, not to be affectionate. This is now a permanent disaster zone. I'm hurt, puzzled, and alone. He withdraws from me at the very time I need some additional support, because I am very sick.

The season draws to a close with a winning record, the best yet: eight wins, five losses, and one tie. The Vikings tie with the Packers for second in the conference. The team seems to be on the ascent, and everyone is anxious for the next season to go even higher. Karl's had a good, steady season and cheerfully looks forward to a vacation from the stress. I'm thinking more about the off-season and what surprises it will hold for me.

‡≈‡ ‡≈‡ ‡≈‡ ‡≈‡ ‡≈‡ ‡≈‡ ‡≈‡ ‡≈‡ ‡≈‡ ‡≈‡ ‡≈‡ ‡≈‡

Chapter 8

Heading Toward Motherhood

$\mathcal{W}$INTER 1965: Karl settles back into his routine of frequent visits to the locker room during the off-season. Once I ask him if he has to work out to keep his muscles in condition, and he says, "I don't spend much time working out off-season. Maybe an hour or two twice a week." Many of the other guys work very hard to maintain their physical condition, but Karl's is mostly natural. As it turns out, working out isn't his only reason to go to the locker room. At Karl's funeral, I will learn there was a long-running poker game in the locker room.

This off-season one of the superfans has given Karl another commission-only job, and I already know this spells very little income for us. The job is selling large installments of chairs for places like schools, auditoriums, stadiums, churches, and convention centers. It involves many meetings, preparation of estimates, and is very time intensive. The competition with other companies is brisk, and Karl doesn't do well at closing the sales, so it will be another entire year with very meager income from the few times Karl receives an honorarium for speaking. Plus my income, of course.

I continue the second quarter of my junior year at the university. The classwork is challenging but stimulating. I find I have an easy understanding of the sciences, and my curriculum is 100 percent science. There are some areas I especially like, such as microbiology, immunology, and anything that has to do with humans.

Around this time I figure out for the first time that I have an eidetic memory, a photographic memory. I have heard many people refer to me as "a mind like a steel trap," that is, after they commented first about my looks. Before now, I never understood that there was something different about the way my mind works.

Eidetic memory can come in a variety of forms. It can literally be seeing in the mind's eye a photograph or page or scene of whatever one turns one's thoughts toward. I could, when I wished, see the actual page in a book or my own notes, including the page number at the bottom, when a question would come up on a test. I used this skill if I didn't easily remember the answer to the question. This kind of memory doesn't help with understanding, though. That's quite another skill, but eidetic memory sure does come in handy on tests.

Eidetic memory can also involve the other senses. For instance, a particular smell can bring to mind every detail of an event that occurred when that smell was last encountered. The same is true for music and sound, even for touch and taste. A professor notices I have this ability by watching how I take tests, and he illustrates it to me through some additional testing. It's a wonderful tool that I haven't understood before. From this point on, I'm able to plan my studying in a very compressed way so as best to utilize this wonderful gift. This is the reason I'm able to get good grades in my classes, in addition to understanding the course work, even though I do very little studying.

Eidetic memory will allow me to navigate my college and medical school studies with relative ease, despite marriage and children. It will be twenty years later, when I suffer a brain injury from an automobile accident caused by a drunk driver, that I will completely lose this eidetic memory. Boy, does that present a challenge then.

For now, Karl leaves every day to be with his buddies and to do his work, and I go to school each day and work in the university research laboratory. These are still very good times in our marriage. We are so much in love. We hold hands all the time and enjoy each other's company very much. We both love to laugh and have fun wherever we go (when he's sober). While Karl is flawed (and who isn't?), he is a good man with a warm heart.

But I can feel the forces slowly gathering that work against a long-term marriage. Our very different backgrounds and upbringings, including our expectations and the working structure of marriage and family, manifest themselves more as the years pass. The pro football arena does not encourage family life, with the exception and expectation that wives will stabilize their husband. Otherwise, families are clearly viewed as an impediment as far as football is concerned and kept out of the way as much as possible. There are very few family gatherings, picnics, or parties sponsored by the Vikings over the years, with almost no nods to the importance of family.

Alcohol and, in time, drugs will continue to create distance between Karl and me, and then there will be the women. I have sensed all this and already realize I'll be unable to alter the course of things. Karl will not discuss any problems, preferring instead to laugh and walk away. And so already in the second year of our marriage, our times together begin to take on a bittersweet flavor for me, because I fear our future. So I savor for now the many good and special times we do have.

†ⱌ†

IN THE second quarter of my junior year, my pregnancy becomes more of a problem. I develop diabetes and preeclampsia (elevated blood pressure with massive swelling of the legs) and am severely anemic, which does not respond to increased iron intake. All of this makes me feel miserable most of the time, and it becomes clear to me that I'm not going to make the third quarter this year. My baby is due in June, but I'm probably going to have to finish the second quarter, and then go to bed rest. This also means I'll get out of sync with the med tech curriculum and will have to wait until next year's spring quarter to swing back into school. I'm not happy about this, but nothing can be done about it. I'm not well enough to continue school and work after the winter quarter.

Meanwhile, Karl and I enjoy our times together. We have a fun time at the Como Park Zoo one day in late winter. At this time, the zoo is very small and very cozy. Visitors can be just twelve inches from the cages, kept back by a flimsy iron railing that anyone can easily reach over. The main attraction is a big gorilla, sitting and taking in the attentions of the visitors who pass by his cage. He doesn't move. He just watches everything with interest.

Then we come to the panther's cage. He's relaxing at the back. For some reason, we lock eyes, and he becomes very interested in me We keep looking each other in the eye, and then, very slowly, he gets up, never taking his eyes off mine. He casually makes his way to the front of the cage, continuing to stare at me. He's just twelve inches from me now, and I'm stunned by his sleek beauty. Then, just as casually, he begins to turn to walk to the back of the cage again. Still, he keeps his eyes on me. Suddenly, he sprays me with extremely pungent panther piss. I've been marked! I'm now part of his territory, and I reek. Karl and many other bystanders are rolling on the ground, laughing. The panther appears quite satisfied with himself and regally returns to his resting spot at the back of the cage.

I'm actually flattered to be chosen by this panther, though the stink will never leave the clothes I'm wearing. They are a permanent loss. And I am laughing right along with everyone else. I watch him a bit longer, then we move on, given a wide birth by the rest of the visitors who smell me. In the future I will miss these days at the Como Park Zoo, because, of course, the zoo is eventually updated to be much safer—as in not getting too close to the animals.

Though our social life revolves mainly around Vikings families, we spend some evenings with my classmates, and our friend R and his wife continue to be in our lives. R tries to be alone with Karl as much as possible, and Karl continues to be clueless about his intentions. I attempt to help Karl open his eyes, but he doesn't believe it and laughs me off. I do enjoy the company of R and his wife. They're funny, creative, dynamic people with a very interesting circle of friends, so we keep up with them. But there is some deep secret in R's past. It's often hinted at, but no one will mention the details, and I can feel the constant very dark energy around him.

This off-season Karl and his Vikings buddies form a traveling basketball team and play exhibitions with local teams throughout Minnesota and neighboring states to earn a few extra dollars. They have a grand time and are often gone for several days on road trips. I don't see many of these games because most are far away, and the wives generally are not invited. Karl seems to be having a good time, and I'm grateful for the occasional one hundred or two hundred dollars added to our resources.

In the middle of my pregnancy and the busy off-season, our new home is gradually taking shape in Burnsville. Of course, the usual construction delays occur: there's too much snow, the contractors have too many houses under construction, and so on. The roadway is unpaved, and when the ice and snow melts, it becomes a quagmire. I'm still hoping for the May move-in date, but it's starting to look a bit too optimistic.

Finally, the winter quarter ends at school, and I will have to take a year's hiatus from my studies until I can get well from this pregnancy and then catch up with the med tech courses provided in the spring quarter. I also stop working until after the pregnancy. I'm supposed to be at bed rest now, but I have too many tasks to do related to the building of our home. And I'm still playing in the orchestras and singing in the choir at church each Sunday, with a Wednesday night rehearsal as well.

Because of the swelling in my legs and body, I will ultimately gain forty pounds with the pregnancy, but I am tall and do not look particularly fat or have an unduly large tummy, and I am able to move about as needed. So when Karl is home, we focus on keeping the house building on track. We often visit the site.

+〜+

Our new home sits on a cul-de-sac at the end of 129th Street in Burnsville. There are no other homes nearby as yet, and the views from the large one-acre lot are quite amazing. We are easily able to see the entire cityscape of downtown Minneapolis and its skyscrapers. Nearby is a drive-in theater with the screen pointed our way, so we will have years of summer entertainment by watching silent movies on the drive-in screen from our living room. Interstate 35 West, a new freeway a few miles away, can be seen out the left side of our living room window. Each night at rush hour the scene becomes an intriguing string of white headlights and red taillights that remind us of Christmas tree decorations. The traffic noise doesn't reach the house, and the silent show is quite delightful.

On one of our spring visits to the construction site, when I am beginning to despair that the house will be finished in time, we pick our way for two blocks toward the house down a muddy mess that will eventually be a paved road. I can see from the top of the hill that no one is working at our house today, and I'm angry, since they're far behind where they should be in the construction. As Karl and I move toward the house, we work hard to stay out of mucky trouble in the mud, but it's impossible.

Suddenly, near our house and without any warning, I break through the mud and fall through a hidden opening. It seems the sewer has been dug and placed—but not the sewer cover. The whole area has been covered over with snow and mud during the winter. I had not seen this and drop into the hole so quickly I haven't the wits to be scared. I have no idea what's happening. Just as suddenly, however, I stop, stuck at my pregnant abdomen in a sea of mud. I don't hit the solid bottom—I have no idea how deep this hole is—so my feet are flapping free in the underground air. I'm starting to have trouble breathing because of the constriction on my tummy and momentarily panic.

But it's such a funny picture that we both laugh at the ridiculous scene, even though I'm a bit scared about getting out safely. I don't know if I could fall further and completely disappear into the bowels of the earth, and I really have no idea how to get out. There is nothing at all to grab on to except Karl.

Karl starts to tug and pull on me. His hands are in my armpits, but he can't get the right grip, and I'm struggling. Finally, because of his great strength, he's able to lift me straight up out of the hole. By this time we look like two pigs that have been frolicking all day in the mud. Only our eyes show through the mess, and we laugh and give up trying to avoid the mud for the rest of the trip to the house. Fortunately, the floors there are still all bare subflooring or concrete, so a little mud doesn't matter.

Getting home in the car is another matter. We get it really dirty with mounds of mud on the floor, seats, and steering wheel. And of course we run into some Viking friends as we try to sneak quietly into our apartment building. They hoot, and before the week is out we are known as the mud king and queen.

⁘

AT THE same time as my pregnancy, my cat Mrs. Plato (also known as Missy) is also expecting a litter of kittens. This is her first. She has matured enough for Plato to finally impregnate her, so our little apartment is full of two pregnant females.

Plato and Mrs. Plato sleep in the crook of my right arm each night. They can cuddle in this way because I am a very still sleeper, rarely changing position even once during the night.

At two o'clock in the morning of May 26, 1965, I am awakened by a disturbance with the cats. They're moving more than usual. When I look to the usual spot in the crook of my arm, there is a new family. Four perfect Siamese kittens—nearly pure white—are nursing at Missy's tits, with Plato sitting watch. I swear he looks proud.

Just as this is registering with me, I turn to Karl to awaken him and tell him the news. As I twist, there is an audible loud pop. I both feel and hear it. And I'm suddenly drenched with water from my pregnancy. So there will be yet another birth today.

I've always thought that my water broke two weeks early because I ate nearly a whole watermelon the day before. The weather had been hot, and the watermelon was cold and tasty. In much later years, when asked by my patients how to get their labor going, I will half-jokingly say, "Try eating a whole watermelon. Sometimes it will make your water break." And it often worked!

At any rate, we must leave the little cat family on its own. I get dressed, and we call Dr. Stromme and head for Abbot Northwestern Hospital near downtown Minneapolis. Delivery is not imminent, so we settle in for a long day of labor. I think it's a good thing I didn't try to finish the third quarter of school; I wouldn't have made it. The quarter would have had three weeks to go, and I wouldn't have been able to complete final exams.

Dr. Stromme is the first doctor in the area to have fathers present throughout their wife's labor and delivery, even in the delivery room. This is revolutionary, as dads have never been allowed in the delivery room, and Karl will be one of the first men to participate in this way.

It seems to me that the labor progresses slowly, and it isn't any fun at all. I've had no prenatal classes or preparation. The idea of classes to jointly prepare expectant parents with the skills for the huge job of labor and delivery is many years yet in the future. Unprepared, I am stunned, shocked, and jolted by the force and pain of the contractions. It's unreal that anything could hurt so much or that anyone would voluntarily put themselves in this position! I hold my breath against the agonizing pain, something that will later be proved as the wrong thing to do. It's much better to breathe large.

The nurses administer something to me called "twilight sleep," a standard medication at this time for pain relief during labor, and it helps me rest between the contractions. But each new contraction jolts me wide-awake with agony, and I grit my teeth rather than complain or scream. I can hear women screaming in other rooms, and I'm determined to be quiet.

Finally, after I have pushed and pushed for two hours in the afternoon, Dr. Stromme informs me that our baby is occiput posterior. This is not a good position for a first baby and is the cause of at least half of all cesarean sections in first deliveries. Normal delivery position causes the baby's head and body to exactly fit the curve of a woman's pelvis, allowing for a smooth outward trajectory. This normal position has the baby entering head first, stage center, face down toward the back of the woman.

But in occiput posterior, the baby comes out face up. This position is exactly opposite the normal curve of the pelvis, so it is quite difficult to deliver, especially on a first delivery, before the tissues have had a chance to be stretched.

It also doesn't help that our baby seems to have a very solid head, like a bowling ball, which does not mold during the labor (gradually get more pointed to fit through the tight areas of the pelvis). This combination of solid head and occiput posterior makes the labor basically arrest, with no further progress. Nevertheless, ongoing severe contractions and mighty pushing continue. Karl rings my hands, rubs my back, hugs me, and actually pushes along with me. I'm afraid he'll get hemorrhoids. I myself will have bloodshot eyes for days after delivery from all the pushing.

We've been moved to the delivery room, and Dr. Stromme announces he'll need to use midforceps to deliver this stubborn little one. Karl's eyes widen with shock and fright as the forceps are produced. They look like giant salad tongs made of stainless steel. His concern worsens as the forceps disappear up to the end of the handles into my body, about twenty inches, and clamp onto the head of the baby. Dr. Stromme sees how pale Karl is and says, "Listen, Karl, there are already two patients here. We won't be able to pick you up off the floor if you faint, so get control of yourself now, please."

With the next contraction, Dr. Stromme pulls—with no results. He struggles and pulls some more—no results. He's pulling me clear off the table. I have to use the handles just to keep myself from falling off the end, and it feels like my insides are being ripped out of me. It will be many years later when I have cancer before I again know suffering to equal this pain.

I think Karl is surely going to faint. His color is now green. He's probably more scared than he's ever been in his life. Watching this painful and brutal struggle to get his firstborn out of his beloved wife is something quite different from chasing down a man twice his size, making a flying tackle, and wrestling him to the ground while simultaneously prying the ball from his arms. This is his wife and baby, and he's trapped in this drama that really looks damaging and dangerous, which it is to my body.

Finally, Dr. Stromme braces his feet at the base of the delivery table and leans backward with all his weight on the forceps while he pulls with all his strength. His grunts are the only sound in the room. I'm pushing too, and pretty oblivious to the pain now as this looks like a possible life-or-death struggle going on. Twilight sleep or not, I'm fully aware of what's happening.

Then this eight-pound-one-half-ounce little boy finally begins to move on out and is delivered faceup around 5:00 p.m. on May 26, 1965. He's mad as hell and squalls immediately. He is red in the face, his nose is smashed flat, and he has a thick head of reddish blond hair. He's vigorous, but I'm torn to shreds. After the placenta is delivered, the next two hours are spent repairing the damage.

Karl is ecstatic. I'll never again see him so completely filled with joy and emotion. Tears fill his eyes. He's thrilled, grinning, proud. He and I have created his first son, his boy! A son! A son! His son! A beautiful boy, though that's a matter of debate right now as he looks like he's been run over by a steamroller. He is obviously healthy and already seems to have the prominent musculature of the Kassulke men. His head is perfectly round, not pointy like all the other babies in the nursery, but he sure does have a beat-up nose! It will take a few weeks for his nose to pop into some recognizable shape.

We decide immediately on the name Kurt Alan Kassulke. (Alan is the name of my brother who was killed in a car accident when he was twenty-seven.) There is a problem, though. As Karl and I examine Kurt's fingers and toes and wonder in awe at this little newcomer, we think his very bowed legs are just another Kassulke trait repeated down the generations. But with further checking, I can see it isn't just his legs. He has clubfeet.

Kurt's feet are sharply twisted, with the front being pulled down, the heels pulled tight in an upward position, and the curve in his feet is severely to the middle. I will learn later in my doctoring years that this situation is most common with first babies—in the absence of other genetic syndromes—and is probably the result of a womb that resists stretching as the baby grows, causing undue cramping of the limbs. I will also learn that it could have been much worse, though at this time

I'm very worried because I'm not a doctor yet, and I don't know the future for Kurt's legs.

Dr. Stromme assures us that Kurt's clubfeet are fixable, probably with casting and not surgery. So we are relieved and relax in that unique and unrepeatable glow that follows a successful pregnancy and birth. Karl is reluctant to leave me when they take Kurt to the nursery, and the nurses want me to rest. Karl takes me in his arms and holds me like the most valuable treasure on earth. He thanks me over and over for giving him such a wonderful son. We are both very emotional. These are truly precious moments that will never again be repeated in our lives together.

Chapter 9

Football Mom

KURT HAS been delivered after quite a struggle. I always will imagine he had very long fingernails and just dug in, not wanting to come out at all. But the forceps won the argument.

Once I'm placed in my hospital room for the postpartum stay, I discover my roommate, Nancy, has had her first baby, a little girl, by cesarean section the day before. She is jolly and laughs with me constantly, and we become fast friends for the rest of our lives. We have a great time from morning until night. We're both still very young, and this seems like an all-night party, with pain added. The nurses have to come in during the nights to make us quiet down, we're having so much fun.

We're both able to laugh and joke at our sagging bellies and other indignities pressed upon us by our postpartum situation. One man who is standing beside me at the viewing window in front of the nursery, turns to me and asks, "When is your baby due?" He's mortified when I point to Kurt. I guess my belly has a way to go before it's flat again.

Nancy and I are very sore, she in her tummy and I in my bottom, so we giggle at the funny way we move when we're out of bed. We admire each other's babies. They are, without a doubt, the most amazing children ever born. Years later, Kurt will go to the prom with his hospital nurserymate. Karl's visits are infrequent and must conform to hospital visiting hours, which are brief on the maternity ward. Nancy's husband is around a bit more because he's a hospital administrator, so he knows how to bend the rules.

Our room completely fills up with flowers from well-wishers, some of them Vikings fans I've never met. Kurt's birth has been announced on the sports page of the *Minneapolis Star Tribune*. I groan inwardly because I'll have to write a lot of thank-you notes, a chore my mother firmly implanted as the correct course of action when a person receives a gift or a kindness. And doctors, nurses, and hospital personnel stop in and introduce themselves to the Vikings wife, so our laughter is often interrupted by a stranger's wanting to peek into our room.

Despite the fun Nancy and I are having, I'm discharged home on the third day after delivery. Dr. Stromme believes a woman and her baby should not stay in the hospital for an entire week after childbirth, which is the standard at this time. He is correct in noting that complications, specifically postpartum and baby infections, will increase the longer a woman stays in the hospital, and he believes recovery at home is just as efficient. In the future he will be proven so correct that hospital stays eventually become just twenty-four hours for a labor, delivery, and postpartum.

So Karl and I take Kurt Alan Kassulke home to our little one-bedroom Bloomington apartment, now filled with two cats, four kittens, a new baby, and us. We're both so in awe of this new little person. It's just amazing that we created him. We gaze at him for hours.

My parents are on their way from Boone to stay with us and to help with the new baby. This is the tradition at this time. Often the grandparents will stay for four to six weeks after a birth. I'm grateful for Mom and Dad's enormous help, since I'm in a lot of pain whenever I move. Those forceps left behind some big tears that were sewn up with stitches that will dissolve over the next few weeks.

It's such a help that my parents are there, but we are surely crowded in that apartment. I'm furious our new house isn't finished on time. It would have made our lives so much more comfortable. I have already learned that very few plans go as imagined, and I've become pretty flexible. "Que Sera, Sera" is a popular song right now, and this is how I approach life these days: whatever will be, will be.

Kurt is a very calm and easy baby. He basically eats (a lot) and sleeps about twenty hours a day. He grows very rapidly. His pediatrician is Dr. Mildred Schaffhausen, a true pioneer woman in medicine who's been in practice for many years. Of course, all of the Vikings take their children to her (we all see the same doctors). The initial concern with Kurt is to get his legs and feet straightened. Dr. Schaffhausen's husband is a pediatric orthopedic specialist, so we take Kurt to see him when he is just two weeks old.

Thus begins a four-month treatment plan to get Kurt's feet and legs straight. I must take him to the orthopedist every two weeks. At each visit the doctor places a leg cast (from his toe tips to just below his knees) on both of his legs. The casts are created in such a way as to place opposing pressure on the various curves and tight spots, so that as growth occurs, bones and ligaments will eventually straighten out and lengthen, and the curve in his feet and legs will gradually disappear.

The casts are tight, and they obviously hurt Kurt, as he whines and cries when they are placed and for a few days after. Then, because he is growing so fast—he will be the height and weight of a three-year-old by twelve months—the bones straighten and the ligaments stretch, and the casts are more comfortable. In two more weeks the old casts, now loose, are removed and new, tight, painful ones are placed. And the cycle repeats itself.

In the meantime, Kurt begins to attempt to move around the floor, and his creative rolling and dragging with those casts on the carpeted floor becomes the subject of many photos and eight-millimeter films. By four months, just as promised, the casts come off for the last time, and Kurt's feet and legs are straight and perfect. He has many sores from the casts rubbing on his baby-tender skin, but they quickly heal.

To complete the treatment, he must wear very uncomfortable shoes for another year. They curve opposite the natural incurve of his feet and are made of stiff white leather, with a tight strap across the top. This is to ensure that his feet stay straight as they continue to grow. Given the genetics he's received from his parents, it's probably predictable that Kurt will grow to become very smart (genius, in fact) as well as a superb, tall athlete (captain of the Stanford wrestling team), gorgeous to look at, and a wonderful musician. He has inherited the very best of both his parents, and straight legs are a good start for his golden future.

⁌⁚⁍

MEANWHILE, THE house is still being built, and it seems like it will never get done. I've informed the contractor that we're moving in at the end of June, finished or not, as we've given notice on our apartment. It's already rented for July 1. Meanwhile, I take Kurt in his little bassinet-carrier when he is two weeks old and drive to the new house with my dad to show him how the construction is coming. It will be dad's first view of the new house.

We still have to walk about a block to get to the house, as the road remains impassable for cars. I am independent and insist on carrying Kurt myself. At the house, the floors are still all subflooring, and much finish work remains undone, but dad can see what the house will be like, and he's so happy for me. We're standing on the cement floor of the ground level room—which will be the family room with a fireplace—talking about all the different parts of the house, when suddenly, the completely unexpected happens.

Without any warning or discomfort, I begin to hemorrhage. The flow of warm blood coming from my womb is such a deluge that it fills my canvas tennis shoes and then creates a spreading pool of crimson on the cement floor before it really registers with me what's happening. My father has no idea what to do—poor man. He's watching his beloved only daughter hemorrhage, maybe to death. There's no phone, and we're more than a block from the car. There are no other houses nearby, and there is no way at all to get help in the face of this truly impressive bleeding.

He does the only thing he can think of to do. He hands me his handkerchief. I don't know what I'm supposed to do with this. Stuff it inside of me? Mop the floor with it? Blow my nose? It's like trying to stop a broken dam with a cork, and despite the seriousness, we both laugh at the absurdity of this handkerchief.

We just stand, looking helplessly at each other as the spreading pool of blood finally reaches a diameter of six feet. Kurt is resting by the door, so he isn't in the blood. I'm getting faint and am not thinking clearly. There's no place to sit down, either. Finally, the bleeding slows, and then stops.

We don't speak. We just stand and wait a moment to be sure it's over. I'm not in good shape. I'm sweating, and the room is going dark. I was anemic before this, and I know what has happened isn't a good thing. I'm very weak and afraid to move for fear of starting the bleeding again or falling. Meanwhile, the blood is soaking into the cement, leaving a giant circle of crimson.

Finally, we walk back to the car, my shoes leaving squishy, bloody footprints all the way. I lean heavily on my dad's arm, while he carries Kurt with the other. I'm not so independent now. I'll always wonder what the workmen thought when they first encountered this red mess of blood on the family room floor. Was someone killed here? But not one construction worker or carpet layer ever mentions it to me. When I get in the car, it is the second time associated with this pregnancy that the car will have to be cleaned after I ride in it. First mud, now blood. My blood-soaked white shorts leave quite an impression.

My dad drops Kurt off with my mom at the apartment, and then he takes me directly to the doctor. It turns out my hemoglobin is so low that I'll have to have some transfusions. So I spend a day in the hospital, filling up my tank, so to speak. And the doctor has to repair a previously undetected torn area of my womb, or perhaps the stitches dissolved too soon. But I'm quickly recovered and want to get home.

Finally, the end of June arrives. Kurt is a little over a month old, and we move to our new house. There is no running water, no gas or electricity, and a haze of dust is everywhere as the workmen sand the woodwork and walls. Toxic varnish and paint fumes fill the rooms. It's an inhospitable place to care for a newborn, but I'm adamant that we live there, or they will never finish it. Work does progress fast once we're watching them daily. I guess the contractors feel guilty when they have to look at us every day.

After we are in the house a few weeks, Karl must leave for training camp. The same rules still apply: wives are not encouraged to come to Bemidji at all. The time away is just as long as before, although Karl will make it home for a few hours a couple of times.

When he is home, he is a loving father, although he does not take any responsibility of any kind in childcare, including feeding or diapers. This is the norm for these years in America: childcare is the woman's responsibility entirely. But Karl loves his son and plays with him on the floor, and they both chuckle and laugh.

After Karl is in camp, many things still need to be finished at the house, and everything seems to move so slowly. Finally we get water and electricity, which eases our problems considerably. The most major item left is to pave the road.

Finally the crews come to grade the dirt down deeply and smoothly in preparation for blacktopping. At this point, our house is essentially finished, including the outside painting, but we still must park our car a block away due to the road.

One day I am in the house, and the crews are working with heavy grading equipment in the cul-de-sac, when I hear a loud clunk. I look out the front window just in time to see a workman in the deep, immense circle that has been graded. Perhaps the cul-de-sac is four feet deep at this point. This workman is bending over, peering at something. He speaks with another workman. They remove their caps and scratch their heads, then make a decision. The first man lights a match and throws it down in front of him.

There is a loud whoosh, and suddenly an eternal flame is burning right in front of my new house, so hot I can feel it inside the house. It shoots up with great force, about fifteen feet into the air. It seems the grader broke the main gas pipe, and the workmen couldn't decide what it was. So they cleverly lit a match, which surely settled the question.

Now the flame is so hot that the new paint on my house blisters and begins to peel off and the wood starts to char. I take Kurt and run up the hill. This doesn't seem like a very safe situation as there's a gas pipe leading directly into my house.

Soon the volunteer Burnsville fire department arrives in the cul-de-sac in a pickup truck, with seven men standing on each side on a specially made platform. They jump off and aim handheld fire extinguishers at the flame, but it's too hot for the men to get close enough. Finally, the flame suddenly disappears. It seems the gas company shut off the main somewhere far away, and that solved the problem.

A representative of the gas company later tells me it was luck that the entire house didn't blow up. I guess I'm comforted by this information. At any rate, the entire front of the house gets new wood and a fresh paint job.

✦◡✦

KARL MISSED all this excitement because he was away at camp. The usual preseason camp is once again full of the regular team plus all the rookies and trades from other teams and free agents (players that have been granted a chance to try out for the team). They all hope to take the job away from a regular player, and some will succeed. Karl's position is no exception, as usual. There are at least two rookies present who are hot for his job. He has more confidence each year, but the danger and risk of losing one's place is always high during camp. And the players' drinking kicks into high gear during this time to relieve the stress.

Karl has already had his humiliating session with the films and Jim Finks. All his errors have been lovingly spliced together, and again none of his heroics make this film. And he accepts another measly two-thousand-dollar raise. By now I know for sure there are players, even on the defense, who are making much more than him, but he's convinced he's just lucky to be playing and wouldn't think of arguing about the small raise. So he'll enter his third year as the starting strong safety for the Minnesota Vikings in 1965 at the spectacular salary of twenty-three thousand dollars.

Another interesting transformation is gradually taking place. When Karl joined the team, it was predominantly white. Each season a few more talented and key black players join the squad (African American is not yet the politically correct reference). The main new players—Carl Eller and Jim Marshall—all seem to blend well, and Karl welcomes these new friends to his circle. All of the years we are there, I am not aware of any significant racism or difficulties on the team, despite many men of the team being southerners. In general, partying together splits more along offense and defense lines rather than color lines. There are many parties with everyone in attendance, and I do not detect any racism. Of course, I can't speak to whatever happens on the field or in the locker room.

Other transformations in America are also gradually taking place. Women's liberation is in its infancy, and there are many jokes about the movement. Burning bras is a big laugh. And the first waves of antiwar protests are beginning to gather support. The young (up to age thirty or so) are embracing the fast-moving hippie culture, although many are just picking up the trappings: colorful shirts and bell-bottom pants, wild jewelry, marijuana, free love, mustaches and long hair, whole food co-ops, pierced ears in women and girls (previously reserved for scuzzballs and women of low reputation), pierced earrings in men (all kinds of rumors abound about this; if in a particular ear, it signals the man is queer—gay is not yet in the vernacular), and the mild rejection of most of the preceding generation's values. Very few are actually living as hippies, most just look like hippies but lead middle-class lives. And the civil rights movement is sweeping the nation as well. These are exciting times for the young, but scary and challenging times for the middle-aged and older.

We begin to hear of other drugs besides marijuana—LSD in particular. Its reputation is very bad, and most of us are frightened to take this drug at all. We've all heard stories of individuals who never are normal after even one dose, and most of my friends and acquaintances, including me, have no interest in taking this risk. I will actually see some of the devastation of LSD in a few years when I am interning. I especially remember a young man who assured his friends he had wings and could fly, then he jumped out an eight-story window and was crushed on the pavement below. Eventually, I will learn that LSD, taken in carefully controlled doses and under watchful support, actually changed many lives for the better. I still will never try it, though. It's just too risky.

The rest of my years with Karl will take place in this ever-increasing sweeping change of mores and ideas about race, women, and the freedom of personal expression. These changes will touch everyone's life, some positively, some negatively. Karl and I are a young couple, not yet sturdy in our maturity, and we are caught in the wild cauldron of celebrity against a backdrop of some of the most sweeping social change seen in America.

For now, I have to figure out how to begin functioning again. It's clear that I prefer working and studying to being home all day, and while Karl is at camp, I find a nearby grandmotherly German woman, Irma, and hire her to be with Kurt each day while I go back to work. She's very special, and I'm comfortable leaving her with Kurt while I work full time.

I'm very excited to get back to my research, which is promising and highly interesting. I've begun to see some of my research papers published in prestigious medical journals, and I am receiving some invitations to present my work at various medical meetings around the country. In the next several years I will present my research at these conventions, but for now my coauthors give the presentations. I feel uncomfortable yet as a first-time mother, and I don't want to leave Kurt when Karl also isn't home.

When I return home from the university each evening, I take Irma to her house—she doesn't drive—then spend the evening feeding Kurt and playing with him. He continues to be a happy, docile guy with a gigantic appetite. It's clear he will be a very big boy and man (six feet four inches when he's finished growing). I am delighted that each visit with the doctor is normal, though he is completely above the growth chart for height, and his weight and head size are exactly proportionate. His only problem is recurrent ear infections, and Dr. Schaffhausen proves to be a truly stunning help in this regard, since every ear infection begins during the night.

I have to be at work at eight o'clock each morning, traversing rush-hour traffic for the more-than-one-hour trip from Burnsville to the university. When I arrive, I park in the flats, several steep blocks below the university hospital, and climb a very long hill to get to the medical school building where my research lab is situated. So it's a good hour and a half to get to work. It's a challenge to get a baby to the doctor and still get to work on time.

Kurt is an unusual child in that he never seems ill and does not cry in pain with his ear infections. His eardrum just suddenly ruptures, so that when I change his diaper, often in the middle of the night, I notice the pus and blood draining from his ear. But I'm able to call Dr. Schaffhausen during the night, and she comes to her office very early, at six o'clock, to see those few sick children who have working moms (still a rarity in these days). After these predawn office hours, which make it possible for me to get to work on time, she goes on to her hospital rounds, then is back in her office until dinnertime. She's quite a role model for me, although I don't know for sure yet that I'll be attending medical school.

And so it goes. I'm back at work and becoming confident in my new role as mother. My health is restored, and my weight is down to very near my prepregnant state. My figure is fine, my belly flat, though scarred with fading stretch marks. The preseason ends with a few wins. There are some promising new additions to the team and some disappearances of other players as well. Karl's relieved that he's still an integral part of his beloved game and team.

Chapter 10

Storm Clouds

*T*HE VIKINGS FAMILIES ARE arriving back in the Twin Cities in preparation for another season. More than half of the team is only in town during the fall. For the rest of the year, they go to their permanent homes. Once everyone is settled in their temporary apartments, the social season and football season begin anew.

The wives resume their bridge games each week, an ongoing source of team gossip, support, and, as I've said, M&M's. To my surprise, there have been no new additions to the group since I arrived in 1963, so we are a tightly knit group, mostly wives of offensive players but one or two defensive players' wives, including me. There certainly are no more rookie wives, as I once was.

There is plenty of gossip: who is caught being unfaithful, who might be taking drugs, who is probably going to be dropped from the team, and who is pregnant. An interesting thing also occurs at the weekly bridge games. Because my field of study includes so much medical information, the women are turning to me with their medical concerns. I know I am hardly the person they should be asking as yet, but we do discuss some of my observations.

For instance, I note that one wife, a delightful woman who has serious and uncontrolled diabetes, also clearly has anorexia. Her body structure is absolutely skeletal; her knee bones are wider than her thighs or lower legs. I talk with her privately about the serious dangers of anorexia, and she cheerfully brushes me off. Later, she will fall while ice-skating and fracture her pelvis. Such a complication should not occur in a young woman. Some years later, she will die young of complications from diabetes and anorexia.

One very funny family event occurs during this season with one of the players who has married the daughter of an alleged crime boss. She is a big woman, taller than me, with big hair, which is the style just now, and a spitfire personality. It soon becomes apparent her very large, strong football husband is probably being physically and verbally abused and is afraid to do anything about it because of his father-in-law. But for now, this couple is a great source of gossip and ongoing discussion. The husband sometimes has a black eye, which is not a common football injury because of the way the helmets protect the face.

Probably my favorite private occurrence of the year (which does not make the newspaper) happens when this couple invites some of the players and families (including Karl and me) to their apartment for an Italian dinner. When the company arrives, there has obviously been a fight, and the husband and wife are not speaking to each other. One visitor excuses herself to go to the bathroom and encounters a very unique scene. Her shrieks of laughter bring us all running.

A large painted Italian porcelain bowl is in shards in the bathtub. On the ceiling, dripping and draping in red strings, seems to be the entire contents of the bowl: spaghetti. It is beyond funny, and the story makes the rounds of the team for the rest of the season. Imagining the scene of this couple fighting in the bathroom and the huge bowl of hot spaghetti thrown at the ceiling sends us all into prolonged laughter every time we discuss it. Of course, this is not a marriage made in heaven, and the football player manages a successful divorce without ending up dead. He is also traded to another team, so this particular slice of life is over, but it sure was fun for the rest of us.

One of the new players is a racehorse of a running back, Lance

Rentzel, drafted in the second round from the University of Oklahoma. The term *racehorse* means a very fine player who is prone to injuries. Lance makes many excellent contributions to the team, but the guys joke about him behind his back because he wears silk underwear. Apparently this apparel is just too over the top for these jocks. But Lance has other problems that will not show up for another year.

We wives all suffer through another cold season under our strange half-sleeping bags, then continue our rounds after each game to whatever celebration has been chosen. Karl has a good season, as usual, but the hopes that the team will continue to improve after the addition of new players gradually disappear when game after game is lost. The final tally will be seven wins and seven losses for the season.

I am more concerned this season, though, about the condition of the guys when they emerge shower-clean after each game. They are fresh and well dressed, but many of them have an unusual glaze to their demeanor, a strange calmness. I ask Karl about it, and he tells me, "We get uppers [amphetamines] before the game. Many of us are taking lots of them, and we need help coming down after the game. So we are provided with downers before we shower. We all feel so much calmer when we take them." Again, he never says specifically who passes out the drugs.

I know we're going to be out for an evening of drinking—I still do not drink alcohol at all—and am worried about the combined effect of these drugs and alcohol. Karl just laughs and says everyone is fine. "Not to worry." But the changes in the guys' postgame demeanor is gradually becoming more obvious each season.

The people around me think it very peculiar that I don't drink alcohol, and whenever we're with other people and wherever we go, I am under constant pressure to drink. No matter what I say or how often I refuse, everyone urges me to drink and brings me all manner of exotic alcohol fruit drinks they're certain I will love. The drinks look pretty, and I take a sip to please them. But whatever the drink, I just don't like the bitter taste of the alcohol and see no reason to drink something I don't like. I confound all the partygoers by simply drinking Coca-Cola. Coke will be my addiction all my life.

⁜

ABOUT MIDSEASON, Karl breaks his right fibula just above the ankle. The fibula is the smaller of the two bones in the lower leg, ending at the outside of the ankle. The normal treatment would be a cast and crutches. But Karl never misses a game or a play. The team trainer expertly tapes the area, stabilizing it, and Karl keeps right on playing. It takes six weeks to heal, and I cannot even imagine the pain Karl feels in this constantly bumped and stressed fracture, but he gets through it without losing his job.

Though he never mentions it, I often wonder if the team is providing him with any narcotic pain medicines, but I will never know. In all our years together, I never see Karl take even so much as an aspirin for pain. Playing football is its own narcotic for Karl, and maybe that's enough. These guys are truly tough in the old-fashioned way. Nothing will stop them short of a broken spine (which is yet to come in Karl's future).

We're still arguing about what that future will look like when the pro football years are over, and the arguments are stronger now. Karl's starting to plan with some other players to buy a restaurant-bar, and he seems to be serious. I still control the funds (at least whatever Karl gives me), and he gives me enough that I know he could never get enough to buy a restaurant from what he's holding back. My real concern about this, besides his drinking, is that he continues to need constant adulation from his fans. He needs it and revels in it, and this adulation has already become more important to him than his family. It has become an addiction as strong as any alcohol or drug.

He will inconvenience or abandon us in any way, in any situation, if it means a fan is stroking his ego. We often drive home alone, without even a good-bye from Karl, who frequently doesn't even notice when we leave. I understand that he loves us dearly and sincerely, but his urges regarding adulation are by far the strongest force in his life. So after two and a half years of marriage, football comes first, then fans, and we are third on his list. When we have him to ourselves, he is an adoring and attentive husband and father. But those times together become more and more scarce as the years pass.

Then, for the first time, a new argument begins. This one involves the purchase of a motorcycle. Some of the Vikings players are beginning to buy motorcycles, big honking Harleys with all the bells and whistles. Karl very much admires this powerful machine. But I'm correctly thinking of his reckless and drunken driving and how very dangerous motorcycles can be, and I refuse him this purchase. This will be an ongoing argument for the rest of our married years—an argument I will win every time until we are divorced.

One more troubling event occurs during the 1965 season. I'm wearing the same clothes I wore before my pregnancy with Kurt, but I'm carrying ten pounds more, though I am still thin because of my height. Quite out of the blue, while undressing one night, Karl comments for the first time ever, "I sure wish you would lose those ten pounds. You look fat."

I'm stunned by this. Karl has thrown this comment off casually and goes right on with his preparations for bed and lovemaking. But I know in my heart that I am now obviously being compared to another woman, or women, who have not borne a child and so are perfect. It doesn't matter that we are a celebrity couple, with very frequent articles in newspapers and magazines and radio and television references to my beauty. I am no longer perfect, and Karl doesn't have to settle for less than perfect. And he probably isn't.

Though we don't discuss it at this time, my intuition tells me that his resistance to the football groupies has ended. It's a heartrending feeling, and I know I can't do a thing about it. Karl is handsome, famous, and fun to be with. He's away from home so often and doesn't need to report his comings or goings. Beautiful women, hungry for his attentions, are a fixture of the scene, wherever he goes. For the first time, I begin to wonder if our marriage will make it.

The season ends in turmoil. The press and the fans are unhappy with the record for the year. Everyone had expected the team to improve, not regress. Fights between Coach Norm Van Brocklin and the media have become a source of consternation for the press and football management and great fun for the public. Van Brocklin is fighting with everyone now, including his quarterback, Fran Tarkenton. This problem escalates during the entire season, and great changes will occur at the end of the season. Van Brocklin will resign as coach, and Tarkenton will ask to be traded. And so Tarkenton leaves for the New York Giants.

Meanwhile, my personal pain at what I feel is surely Karl's infidelity is difficult to handle. It isn't something he's going to talk about, and I know it. I won't discuss it with anyone else for many years. For the first time, I begin to understand my own method of coping with a complicated life. I've become an expert at compartmentalizing my life. Although there is some obvious overlap, I have separate boxes for children, family, marriage, football, work, and my education. Each has its separate requirements and happiness and sorrows, and I find I can just turn off one box and close the lid when I'm in a different area of my life. Of course, football and celebrity can never be completely shut off, as the public doesn't allow it. In general, though, I am able to negotiate this increasingly complicated life with grace, by using these boxes and compartments. I even become aware of them to the point of consciously opening or closing certain areas whenever it's necessary to concentrate on something else.

So our third season of professional football draws to an end. Karl has had another ruggedly good season, and his position seems secure. We all wonder who the new quarterback and coach will be.

Karl still revels in his celebrity, his adoring fans, and his beer. In a way, I am seeing him for the first time as a man-boy who will never grow up and who uses defenses that served him well while he was living in a challenging home. But they are roadblocks that prevent us from ever dealing directly with our own issues. As a couple, though, we've met so many changes in such an overwhelmingly short time.

Now it's December 1965, and I am just recently turned twenty-one. I am a wife of two and a half years, a mother of a seven-month-old baby boy, a university student with two and two-thirds years finished who is gradually becoming a successful scientific researcher, and a homemaker. I have moved five times and built a new home. I have mastered the knowledge of the game of pro football, both the culture and the rules, and watched my husband transform from a relative innocent to a tempted, mood-altered, unpredictable celebrity.

And my period is two months late. I never miss a period. My life is complicated, but I remain an optimist and laugh and smile a great deal. I enjoy most of the moments of my life, but deep in my heart, I do not know if my marriage can survive.

Chapter 11

A Summer to Remember

AFTER CHRISTMAS I PLAN to go to the doctor for a pregnancy test. I'm sure there's going to be another baby, but I haven't told anyone as yet, not even Karl. Then, one night in early January, I begin to feel mild cramps, which worsen as the night goes on. Suddenly, blood gushes again, and the cramps get severe. I phone Dr. Stromme, and he tells me I'm probably having a miscarriage. He advises that I rest and keep in close contact with him, especially if heavy bleeding continues. He asks me to see him in the morning and to save any tissue if I should pass some.

I do indeed pass a clump of material that is clearly not a blood clot, and the cramping and bleeding improve after that. Karl is blissfully sleeping off a night of drinking and is only minimally aware of any of this activity. In the morning I see Dr. Stromme. After he examines me and the bottle of bloody material I've brought with me, he tells me, "You've had a miscarriage. I'm so sorry, but please know this doesn't in any way mean you can't have more children. You're studying perhaps to become a doctor, so you need to know that one in five pregnancies ends in miscarriage. This occurs because of what we call 'a blighted ovum.' This means fertilization of the egg did occur, and it probably did divide a few times, but eventually the part that was to develop into the baby ceases to grow, and the part that is the placenta remains, giving a positive pregnancy test and slightly enlarged uterus."

He continues to reassure me, tells me what to watch for regarding complications, asks me to be sure not to get pregnant for at least three months, and sends me home. It's only when I get home that I tell Karl we have lost a baby. I'm in a kind of quiet shock. He's very upset and leaves to go out with the guys to settle down with some drinking. I sit on the stairs and cry alone.

Years later the percentage of miscarriages will drop to one in four, presumably because of toxins and changes in our environment, though the real reason isn't known. In this same period, infertility in general is on the rise, and male infertility, in particular, has become a serious issue, with the sperm count in males generally dropping dramatically in all groups.

I will always wonder as I learn more about medicine through the years why the term for the cause of most miscarriages is "blighted ovum" rather than "blighted sperm." It's just one of many terms surrounding the care of women that is never questioned. My favorite of these terms is "elderly primigravida." This term means a woman who is pregnant with her first baby at the age of thirty or later.

For me, though, I just have to go on, assuming another pregnancy will come along when it's time. I'm enjoying Kurt as he blossoms, working every day, playing bridge once a week, singing in the choir every Sunday, with Wednesday night rehearsals, and playing in the orchestra. I have plenty to enjoy in my life in my beautiful Burnsville home.

Karl doesn't often attend church with me, though he is there when Kurt is baptized. He does occasionally come with me, but he's actually not even available on Sundays for at least five months out of the year, and I can count on both hands the number of times he attends church in all of our married years.

But the church is well aware they have a celebrity in their midst. Richfield Methodist Church is currently a large, thriving congregation, with a charismatic and kind pastor, George Chant. Male members of the church ask Karl if he and I would consider visitations with them to prospective members of the church. We both agree to do this, and Karl does follow through with me on several visits. Sometimes he goes on his own with the other male members of the visitation group. Karl, of course, is good publicity for the church and does help attract some new members.

The situation with R, however, gets worse during this off-season. He actually persuades Karl to go into business with him in some very vague way. Karl isn't sure what the business is, but as usual, he tries to get an off-season job, and this will be it for this year.

As much as I try, I cannot get R or Karl to be specific about the business, but R is very optimistic about the big money they will make. I am very skeptical and feel quite sure that this is a ploy to be with Karl. Karl doesn't want to even think about any sexual aspect to R's interest. He points out, correctly, that R is a very successful businessman, and I should just trust he would do what's best for Karl.

One day Karl comes home wearing a very expensive suit bought at one of the most exclusive men's stores in Minneapolis. He looks fabulous, but it isn't something we can afford, and I'm upset at this unrealistic expenditure.

He thinks to calm me by saying, "Don't worry. I didn't buy it. R did." This surely does not calm me.

"Do you mean to tell me that R stood in the dressing room with you while you tried on suits?"

"Yes. So what?" Karl asks. As far as he's concerned, it's no different than the locker room.

I know Karl has absolutely no homosexual tendencies, so I am not worried about this in that way, but I try to explain to him that he is actually torturing R with what probably looks to him like an interest in developing a physical relationship. However, Karl is innocently clueless about this, as usual, and refuses to discuss it anymore. I beg him to return the suit because of the encouraging message it sends R, but he will not. "I need this suit to look professional in our business together," he says, and that's that.

One day R sends me another large bouquet of brilliant red roses. There's no particular event or reason for this, and I recognize it as another attempt to get me on his side and keep me there. Another day he presents me with a gift he obtained in the Caribbean. It's a necklace, quite long, made of bones fashioned into a human skeleton. I will not wear this necklace, and it will be many years later before I actually realize this gift was probably a hex or evil spell that R hoped to work on me. I am very suspicious that some of the bones in the necklace are real human finger bones.

One day I will have an expert in voodoo look at the necklace, and he tells me, "Yep, this is a very bad juju necklace. It's meant to bring terrible luck, perhaps even death, to its owner. And yes, the bones are human." I'm horrified and promptly sell the necklace to the expert. I want it out of my house immediately.

The business goes nowhere, of course, and to my knowledge, Karl does not earn any money. But we are wined and dined all season by R and his wife.

A particularly disturbing event occurs during this time, and I believe Karl finally begins to wonder a bit about R and his attentions. Karl tells me he must go to New York with R for a business conference. Again, I have no idea what this business is, not does Karl. But off he goes with R. When they arrive, they check into the hotel, and Karl discovers their room has just one bed. When Karl protests, R smoothly explains that New York is full of conventions at the moment, and this is the only room they can get.

They are supposed to be gone three days, and I am surprised when Karl shows up the next evening, having taken a taxi home from the airport. He will not give any details and only tells me about the one-bed room and that the business meetings had been canceled. That's all I will ever learn about this alleged business, but we see R less often, though he and his wife will remain in our circle of friends for as long as Karl and I are married. And R palpably pines for Karl whenever I see him.

The tragic story about R now begins to unfold. It seems he is an alcoholic who has not had a drink for several years. He stopped drinking right after a tragedy with his young child. I never knew that he and his wife had any children. R had been charged with watching his three-year-old play in their swimming pool. But R was drunk, and the child drowned while he was completely out of it. He stopped drinking immediately, but he will never get over this tragedy, and it will lead to more tragedy in the future.

And now another problem surfaces: R begins to drink again. His descent is so fast that, over the next several years, he will gradually lose his successful business. His wife stays by him, though, and we still see them occasionally, but less and less over time.

⁓

MEANWHILE, THE third quarter at the University of Minnesota begins, and I have started back to school. I am in sync again in my medical technology course, with a different group of people (I'm now a year behind). I will finish my junior year in June.

Part of the course work involves learning how to work in each hospital laboratory: drawing blood, the tests, and the machines. Each lab has a manual to learn and follow, and each student must know how to perform every test done there, both by hand and by machine, as well as manage any machine malfunctions. So there are endless electrical diagrams and functions for me to master.

In this last quarter of my junior year, I will finish the first round of the laboratory stints and the last of the textbook classes. But I already know that analyzing the fluids and excretions of sick people or drawing their blood does not fulfill me. More than ever, I'm determined to become a doctor, but there are still forces in my family—primarily my husband's family—that persist in undermining this dream by scoffing at such nonsense. Karl, though, is beginning to realize I just might become a doctor, and he is not especially resistant to the idea.

The senior year of medical technology has two tracks. The regular course involves rotating again through each of the labs, learning in even more depth the complete management of each lab, as these students will be managing hospital laboratories when they finish their course work. But for honor students (those with high grade point averages) there's a second choice, which must be petitioned for. This choice allows students to spend their senior year doing a research project, with a paper presented at the end of the year to summarize the project. Students who choose this track probably will not be running clinical hospital labs when they graduate. Instead, they will most likely work in research for their career.

Since I'm already well established with my research and working in an exciting lab, I petition for this track and am accepted. So for my senior year, starting in the fall of 1966, I will work full time doing ongoing explorations, and after a school year of this, I will graduate with a bachelor of science degree.

Karl continues his usual off-season pattern of many speaking engagements (mostly unpaid), frequent exhibition basketball games with his Vikings buddies (occasionally well paid), visits to the training room, and frequent drinking marathons in the afternoons and evenings.

This off-season, Karl and I take an NFL-sponsored trip to Hawaii. Many Vikings attend, as well as many players from other teams, whom we all get acquainted with. The trip is fun and very exotic for me. Hawaii is beyond my very limited travel imagination, so I drink in every sight, the balmy weather, and the ocean—my first real view of this amazing body of water. It's interesting to meet so many other NFL families off the field of play, and I see we all have much in common.

Probably my most memorable experience of this trip will be a visit Karl and I make to a greenhouse where orchids are grown. Karl stays outside and talks with friends. He's not especially interested in orchids. I wander through aisle after aisle of these truly exotic blooms. At this time orchids are a rarity in Minnesota, though they will one day be available in every supermarket.

As I am walking down one aisle, a tiny Japanese man, apparently one of the gardeners, approaches me. He takes my hand and motions for me to follow him. We stop in front of a spectacular display of orchids, and the sign in front reads Dendroglia. I don't know anything about orchids, except that they are exotically beautiful.

The gardener takes out a beat-up pair of snips and pulls down a branch containing about twenty beautiful blooms. He snips it off, grins, then presents it to me. I try to thank him. I am so stunned and grateful, as I know what this branch would cost back in Minnesota. He just grins again, pats me on the arm, disappears around the display, and is gone. I will treasure this branch of blooms for my entire Hawaii trip. For some reason, it impacts me more than the volcanoes or the surfers or the thousand other exotic sights and foods on the islands.

Back in Minnesota, I've just finished my junior year at the university and am working full time again for the summer. Kurt is now a year old, and after a very funny time of crab walking on one leg and both arms (he couldn't stand the tickle of the grass on his feet), he is now sturdily walking. He's very good natured, rarely fusses, and is a complete delight. Irma continues to watch him during the day while I work, then I take her back to her home at the end of each day.

Kurt loves to play in the lawn sprinkler and adores his sandbox and his books. He spends hours outside each day, for this is still a time when the simplest things delight a child, such as a stick in wet sand. There are not yet electronic sounds to make babies sleep or electronic games or even many toys that involve electronic sounds. Kurt is exposed a great deal to music, as I often play piano or my classical music recordings. Years later, Kurt, himself an accomplished pianist, will nostalgically request a copy of my score of Bernstein's "Rhapsody in Blue," over thirty pages long and quite expensive to buy. It's a piece Kurt will frequently hear while growing up, as I love to play it on the piano. He will daily sit beside me and enjoy the complex sounds.

✛✛✛

KARL AND I take a few days to visit in Milwaukee. It's more common for Karl's parents to come and see us in Minneapolis, but we decide to take Kurt to see them. Disaster occurs when we are hardly inside the front door of the Kassulke flat. Otto is home early—it's just after lunch. Karl and I had plans for the afternoon, assuming Otto would get home around five o'clock, but now it looks like that may not happen, and I'm disappointed.

Otto insists Karl come with him immediately to the corner bar, where everyone is waiting to greet him. I put Kurt down and remind Karl of our fun family plans—the spectacular Milwaukee Zoo. There will be no other time than now, as we'll only be in Milwaukee for two days.

Otto quickly reddens at my impertinence. He steps in front of me, then actually butts his belly against mine, knocking me backward a few steps! But I'm no longer silent with this nonsense.

"What do you think you're doing? I'm not some bar fight for you."

"Listen here, lady, this is my house. I'm the adult here, and I'll do as I want."

"Well," I say, "if you're the adult, why don't you act like one?"

This wasn't one of our better visits. Karl, of course, went off with his dad, and Kurt and I sat by ourselves until late afternoon, when the rest of the family arrived home.

This summer Karl and I will begin a new kind of travel. We have some new Vikings friends from Duluth who have a huge yacht. It's made of polished wood, is fitted out luxuriously, and makes frequent long trips on Lake Superior. We'll spend at least a week each summer for the next four summers traveling on Lake Superior on this giant boat.

Our friends are lovely and gracious people and good company, and we're grateful to be treated to this new slice of life that neither of us knows much about. The boating life is an exclusive arena, with its own set of rules and behaviors, and we quickly learn the culture in order to fit in on these trips. My favorite new awareness is of the running disrespect between the owners of motorboats (which we are on) and those of sailboats. Each group disdains the other, and I think it's all very amusing.

The first year we depart from Duluth and travel fairly close to the shoreline to the beautiful Madeline Island area. We explore the island during the day on bicycles and are back on the boat each night. From the mooring there, we take day trips on the boat to see many other Lake Superior islands and to experience the curious fogs that hang about ten feet above the still water so that all is clear below the fog. It feels like being completely alone on the planet because of the dense shroud above us.

Of course, we fish for lake trout, which are very large fish, not like the little brook trout I'm used to catching. I need to be taught an entirely new method of deepwater fishing with weighted lines. The sluggish heavy tug that feels like a snag is often a fish on the line, and the lake trout doesn't fight much until it gets nearer the surface. Then it has to be netted as quickly as possible, because that is when it makes its move to get away. I adore fishing, though I will not bait the hooks, as minnows or suckers are used, and somehow that's a bit different for me than worms.

It's an idyll of a trip, only marred by the loss one day of our hostess's giant diamond engagement ring. It seems she tripped on the gangplank getting on the yacht, and the ring fell from her finger into the muck. All the rest of the days we are on Madeline Island, scuba divers will work daily to sift through the thick mud, but it's fruitless. The ring is gone forever, perhaps a harbinger of a marriage that also will one day be gone between these very nice people.

And so the summer quickly turns to training camp time. There's a new development this year. Training camp has been moved to Mankato, Minnesota, so Karl will only be about one hundred miles away instead of five hours by car in Bemidji. He'll be back in mid-September after training camp and the preseason games. He's had his usual shaming talk with the general manager and once again has settled for a two-thousand-dollar raise. The usual two draft choices for his position will be in camp, so he is getting nervous as usual and anxious to get his position cemented. And so the cycle goes.

~~~~~~

Chapter 12

The Growing Storm

ONCE AGAIN, KARL IS getting restless for me to be pregnant. So while he is gone, I visit Dr. Stromme again and learn I have the same easy-to-treat problem as the last time. Once again, he performs the procedure, with the cramps and the acrid smell of burning flesh and smoke rising from behind the modesty sheet. I receive the same instructions: no sex for three weeks. Not a problem, since Karl is gone to camp. And I am told the same as before: "You'll be pregnant in no time."

With that over, I pass the time while Karl is away. Things are going well in camp, and he feels he will keep his job. By now Karl is truly a fixture of the team—a cheerleader and spirit lifter—the "Hunkie" who brings life and joy to the whole team, as well as playing with a ferocity rarely seen. The entire league respects Karl, and I often see pregame mentions of him in the newspapers of the opposing teams. So although the pressure to perform at all times and to never miss a game or play remains the same, both of us are more relaxed about staying perma-nently in our home in Burnsville. It looks like our life will follow this same cycle with the Vikings until Karl can't play anymore. With this season he will surpass the average length of a pro football career (three and a half to four years is an average career), so these are golden years for him now. There is no telling how long he can keep it up, and at age twenty-five, he shows no signs of slowing down.

But there's a very real dark side to his success, not yet understood in 1966. Studies in the 1990s and into the twenty-first century will demonstrate that the average professional football player loses one to three years off his lifespan for every season played. By 2008 the average lifespan of former professional football players is fifty-five years, and that of linemen is fifty-one to fifty-two, more than twenty years less than an average man in America.

Some of the reasons for this are that the players take such a beating, week in and week out, and they eat very unhealthy meals, with diets stressing red meat, fat, and high calories. Probably many have used steroids. By 2008 there is rising concern that the primary reason for the shortened life span of players, besides drugs, alcohol, and diet, is recurrent concussions, and a study is being conducted at Boston University on the life-shortening effects of repeated concussions. By 2008, twenty NFL players have donated their brains to this study. There is even a new medical term for this problem: chronic traumatic encephalopathy (CTE). The effects of CTE usually begin some time later than the injuries, perhaps even years. They include memory loss, impulsivity, depression and suicide, poor judgment, risk taking, and neurological deterioration that can lead to death.

One researcher commented that the best way to preserve the lifespan of football players would be to wear no helmet at all. Then they would not bang their heads with such ferocity—or so the researcher thought. Knowing Karl, I think he would have banged his head just as hard, helmet or not. The researchers are forgetting the powerful drive these guys have to pound their opponents into the ground. They live to hit, period. And they pay a huge price for it. Karl never earned much money, but even the millions NFL players earn by 2010 isn't really enough to compensate them for the loss of twenty or more years of their lives.

At any rate, this preseason Karl will be escorted home from Mankato three times by the highway patrol. They help Karl to the front door, and they tell me each time, "He's obviously drunk and was going a hundred miles an hour, ma'am. He probably shouldn't drive for a few hours." There is no suggestion of a warning ticket or a citation. These are the days when celebrities and sports figures are protected in general from problems with the law, whether these involve alcohol, drugs, or sexual misadventures. So there are few penalties or any help for problem behavior. The same is true for the teams: there are no drug-testing programs and no warnings about drug or alcohol abuse. As far as I know, this is many years before steroid abuse becomes a problem.

Karl seems to be getting drunk on his free day each week before heading home from camp, then driving one hundred miles an hour up Highway 169 to see his wife and son. More than once, my heart is filled with cold feelings of dread for Karl's well-being. He is too reckless, too sure that life will take care of his devil-may-care activities, living too much on the edge. When I think about my marriage lasting, I fear Karl himself might not last just as much as I worry about the women he's probably messing with.

✦

KARL LIKES the new coach, Bud Grant. Over the next few years, Grant will lead the team to many more victories and much more stability. With a personality the polar opposite from Van Brocklin's, Grant is calm and cool, measured in his reactions, and very analytical. He's fair and brings a strong intellect to the game.

The new quarterback, after some wrangling for the position in training camp, turns out to be a darkly handsome man named Joe Kapp. He also is a polar opposite of Fran Tarkenton. Tarkenton's frantic scrambling to get rid of the ball when he was in trouble is replaced by Kapp's measured and apparent calm control, usually following the prescribed play as it was designed to be executed. Many years later, Kapp will be the head football coach at USC when Kurt is working on his master's degree in film there. It is a very small world, indeed, something I discover nearly daily.

Joe's wife, Marcia, is a beauty who's actively pursuing a career as a model. She and I will be friends and will have some adventures together in the future. Along with many of the recognizable couples on the team, like Karl and me, Joe and Marcia quickly become media darlings. Sometimes the articles are just about Marcia and me, without the men.

I'm working full time, and faithful Irma still safely watches Kurt each day. She is very old, with a German accent, and Kurt is happy with her and doesn't cry when I leave for work. Things at work are getting interesting as well. Soon I will begin my senior year, but I will actually be working in the same laboratory the entire three quarters. I have to prepare my proposal for the exact research project I will do, as well as how I plan on going about it.

I decide I'll work with cell surface membranes in an attempt to identify, if possible, an antigen (identifying landmark) that somehow is not expressed or has become hidden, thus allowing cancer to grow, since the body would not notice it under these circumstances. The work will involve immunology and has overlapping questions and consequences with the new field of organ transplantation and rejection, so it's a hot topic. Researchers all over the world are approaching the question from many different angles.

My proposal not only is accepted, but I receive a large grant (forty thousand dollars) to do the work. This allows me to have a space in the laboratory for myself. I can also get the expensive materials and equipment I'll need, including the radioactive isotope tritium. The grant even allows me to hire an assistant. She proves invaluable, and I'm able to continue the research all the way through medical school, thanks to her diligence. All I have to do is devise the experiment and give her instructions to carry it out. Then she follows it perfectly, and I'm able to trust her results completely.

Another woman, Bernice, is working in the same laboratory and doing research in a similar area. She has her master's degree in medical technology, so technically she has a higher pay scale than I and a higher place in the pecking order, but my grant is better than hers. Though we have worked in the same lab for three years, I begin to detect a bit of jealousy toward me. Some of her remarks are quite sharp. For now, I just let them go by. In the future, the situation will become dangerous, but I have no clue about this just yet.

Each night Kurt and I play, then he sits quietly beside me on the piano bench as I practice my favorite piano pieces—anything Bach and "Rhapsody in Blue" and Dave Brubeck's "Take Five." He already has, at eighteen months old, a quiet intensity when he is observing things. He takes in everything and grows in words, speech, and understanding at a breathtaking speed.

He loves reading books with me but is impatient with this process, as no one can read to him 24/7. So by age three he will have taught himself to read, and by six he will have read every book in sight. That will be his pattern throughout his growing years. He cannot get enough to read.

If he has any problem during these childhood years, it is that he is tall and muscular, so some of his teachers will expect more maturity from him than is reasonable. While he will be at the twelfth grade level intellectually by seventh grade, he is still just a twelve-year-old in his social development, and I have to constantly remind his teachers of this. I remember what it was like to always be the tallest, and there are similarities for him in this way.

For now, though, he is our wonderful little boy. He is good-natured like his dad and loves to play with us, with other kids, and by himself. He looks like a blond version of his dad. While Karl has black hair and a dark complexion, Kurt has my coloring, with reddish blond hair. But comparisons of his baby pictures with his dad's show that other than their coloring, they could be twins.

We have new neighbors now. A house has been built next door, to our left, and Jim and Karen will be our lifelong friends. As it turns out, they will be among the very few who are true and remain in my life after Karl and I split. We freely stop in to chat with one another, and it's nice to have them nearby, although I am an introvert and don't seek out constant companionship.

I am learning that I need space—lots of it—and this house in Burnsville, built in a completely empty area, will gradually become surrounded by houses and other developments as Burnsville grows to be the second largest city in Minnesota. At first it's refreshing to have wonderful neighbors, but I quickly learn that not all of the newcomers are wonderful. Some of them will prove to be jealous of us, and others will frown on of my working and going to medical school (women still are mostly homemakers). Those who disapprove make sure I'm aware of their feelings. This kind of behavior makes my butt tired! I find I have no time for such nonsense and resolve to live farther out in the country when I can.

⌁

DAILY LIFE goes on in this, by now, very familiar cycle as the days pass before the end of preseason. The preseason games are promising, the new additions to the team seem to be adding some depth to the roster, and the season ahead looks very positive. Karl will clearly make the team, and some of the previous players will be traded to another team or just fade back into regular life. Soon the guys are home from camp.

One September morning we open the newspaper to a startling article in the sports section. Lance Rentzel has been arrested for exposing himself to two girls. What a shock! It's the first time I have seen any misbehavior of the team end up in the news. Apparently this one just couldn't be ignored. Lance is clearly disturbed. He will agree to psychiatric care and is let off with a disorderly conduct charge.

After the season ends, Rentzel is traded to the Dallas Cowboys. There he seems to find a home, plays well, and in 1969 is married to Hollywood starlet Joey Heatherton. Everything crumbles again in 1970 when he once again exposes himself. He authored a book about all this: *When All the Laughter Died in Sorrow*. I never saw Lance after his disastrous last year with the Vikings. With all the manly sexual behavior going on around football players, I can only imagine the endless comments Lance received in the locker room.

Once the season starts, the same routine comes back: the drugged postgame behavior, the drinking with buddies up and down the establishments along I-494, the excitement and tension of the games, the separation every week for one to three days before the games.

One Thursday the guys leave in the morning to fly to a game in Los Angeles. They will have the day to rest when they get there, then practice Friday and Saturday in the stadium before the game on Sunday. I leave for the university just after Karl's gone. It's a struggle to get to work due to a very heavy fog hanging over the city. Traffic is backed up, and I'm an hour late just getting to the university. At the end of the day, I struggle in the gloomy dusk to get home. The fog has worsened, and visibility would be zero were it not for the headlights shining through the dense miasma. After ninety minutes, I finally arrive home, then bundle Kurt and Irma in the car to get Irma to her house. When Kurt and I get back home, it's already seven o'clock and quite dark out.

Just when I get in the door, the phone rings. It's one of the wives of the bridge club calling to confirm the next bridge date. While we speak, I say, "Isn't that Milt I hear in the background?" She says, "Yes, the guys didn't leave this morning. The airport's closed due to the fog. Why, isn't Karl home yet?"

Karl is not here yet, nor has he even called to let me know they didn't leave. I'm just flat out pissed! I know he's with his buddies, drinking and doing whatever else on the I-494 strip. But it's very foggy out, and I'm worried about him driving drunk in this weather. I decide to try to find him and fetch him safely back.

But there's a code among the bar owners and restaurateurs regarding queries from wives. They all lie and say, "He was here, but he left x number of hours ago." I follow this trail of lies through several establishments. I'm sure he's in one of them, but they will not put him on the phone.

Midnight comes, and still no call from Karl. He's now been drinking from about ten o'clock in the morning, when the flight was canceled, and not a word from him. So I decide to get even. I'm fed up and worried sick, but there's nothing I can do but hope he gets safely through the fog.

At this time we don't ever lock our doors. We don't even carry keys, which means if I lock the doors, Karl will be unable to get in. I lock all the doors.

At two o'clock in the morning I'm awakened by someone pounding on Kurt's bedroom window, which is on the second level above the garage. "Janny!... Janny!... Let me in!" Karl has picked up Kurt's huge sandbox, dumped out all the sand, and tipped the sandbox on end. Even in his drunken state, he's able to climb up on the wooden sandbox, and from there onto the garage to reach Kurt's window.

I pick up the phone and call the police. "Please come quick! My husband is gone for an out-of-town game, and there's someone on my garage pounding on my windows. Please, hurry!"

When the police arrive, they pull down a very sheepish Karl from the garage roof, and then knock on my door to let them in. They lead Karl in, and I feign surprise that it's him. "What's going on? You're supposed to be in Los Angeles!" So he has to explain in front of the police what he's been doing all day and that he didn't let me know that he was still in town.

I'm so angry I don't speak to Karl and just go back to bed. I have to get up and go to work in the morning. He goes into the bathroom to vomit, then falls asleep on the bathroom floor, where I leave him (it's carpeted). What a change this is from the first few times he came home and vomited. How I cared for him, cradled his stinking head, wiped the toilet clean. That's all over now, though. I've had enough.

In the morning I leave without speaking to him, and he then departs for Los Angeles. But my revenge isn't yet complete. I have hair that tumbles to below my butt, and Karl loves it very much. So I make an appointment for Saturday with the hairdresser and cut off all my hair into something called a Sassoon cut. This is very short hair all over my head, with pointy wisps of longer hair in front of my ears. I look great with it, but like another person. I save the cut-off hair and have a beautiful curly hairpiece made from it. I will wear it on the back of my head whenever I wish to dress up.

And I'm still not finished. I go to an exclusive favorite clothes shop in the Hennepin-Lake shopping area, Schlamps, and find a gorgeous blue suede long coat with a gray fox fur collar. It isn't something I would usually buy because of the expense—$250—but today I'm going to buy it. The coat turns out to be my favorite for many years, but right now it's a luxury I believe I've earned and will have if I wish.

So on Sunday night the new me, with my wonderful coat and short hair, arrives at the airport to pick up Karl after the Los Angeles game. He actually flirts with me as he passes by but does not recognize me. I have to run after him and catch him. "Karl!... Karl!... It's me! Your wife! Remember me?"

He can't believe his eyes. He doesn't know how to react. His face is like a fast-forward video, with so many emotions running by it's hard to figure where he'll stop. Finally, he focuses on me again, and it's clear he completely understands what has happened. Something very fundamental has changed here. Finally his behavior has caused me to do something drastic, and he is very, very sorry.

"Janny, I'm so sorry. I was so stupid. Please forgive me? Please, please forgive me. I know it was wrong. I'll never do it again. I promise. You'll never have to worry again. Please, I love you so much. Buy all the coats you want. Buy a mink coat! I love your hair! I just didn't recognize you. You're so beautiful! How could I make you worry so much... I'm so, so sorry. Please, please forgive me."

All of this is taking place at the airport concourse while the other players and their wives are passing curiously by. Many of them don't recognize this new glamorous person, either. Of course I will forgive Karl. I love him and am now thoroughly codependent, though it will be many years before I understand this term that describes how behavior changes occur in those who love an alcoholic or addict. So though these words are an echo of similar words I heard when we were just courting, and circumstances have become so very much more severe in this alcohol arena, I will forgive him, and we will go on. But it has been another nail in the looming coffin of our marriage.

And so the season continues, with the team actually going backward in their record. They win only four games, lose nine, and tie one. The media chalks it up to a new coach and a new quarterback. Next year will be better.

Despite the major upset in our marriage, our social life and media attention progress as if nothing has happened. But it has happened, and I think this is truly the time when I begin to think about another life, one without Karl. It's very painful, though, and I don't take any action. I'm pretty sure the future does not hold any golden wedding anniversary celebrations for us.

And at the end of December, I miss my period again.

Chapter 13

Ups, Downs, and More Ups

*K*ARL TAKES OVER THE management of the Vikings exhibition basketball team this off-season. The guys are having a blast. Teams all over the five-state area challenge them for a fun game. It's not so easy beating the football players (many are multitalented in sports), and sometimes these teams are poor losers. I never hear these stories, but Ron Pitkin, the coauthor of Karl's book, tells me in 2010, "One of the games nearly turned into a riot when a player on the opposing team showed poor sportsmanship, and one of the Vikings knocked him flat halfway up the bleachers."

The Vikings have fun, but they take winning seriously. And this activity brings in some funds, so Karl throws himself into it big-time and is one of the team clowns. Unfortunately, sometimes Karl forgets to line the team up for a scheduled game, and then he has some very irate fans. He expands his arrangements to include scheduling speaking engagements for the team and also forgets to send the guys out from time to time. When they don't show up for a big evening somewhere out of state, I hear Karl on the phone trying to explain his oversight—both to the Vikings who didn't get informed and to the activities chairman of these various events. Sometimes I have to take the calls, since Karl isn't even home but is out drinking somewhere.

Karl picks up the ringing phone. "Oh, hello there, Tom. How's it hanging today? Honk, honk!"

Silence. Karl listens for a while, then says, "You must be mistaken. I couldn't have forgotten a game tonight. In Fargo? No way. I'm sorry, Tom, but you must have put the wrong date on your schedule."

Silence again, then, "Well, I'm sure sorry about those five hundred folks who bought tickets for tonight, but you just got the date wrong. Guess that's a whopper, huh? Honk, honk!"

Silence, then, "Well, sure, I can check my book, but I wouldn't forget something so important. That would be awful rude. Just a minute."

After he checks his book, his voice has lost its bounce. "Well, by golly, you're right! We do have you on the schedule. Wait, Tom, well, wait a minute—."

By now I can hear Tom screaming on the other end of the line.

"We'll just come another day. I don't see what's the problem. Just pick another date and everyone can come then, right?... Tom? Tom? Huh, I guess he hung up."

Of course, the biggest deal for the players is to hang around, sign autographs, and schmooze after the games. Their most exciting game this season is with the Harlem Globetrotters, and quite oddly, the game takes place in the high school auditorium in the little suburb of Shakopee, so I get to watch it. It's always entertaining to watch the Harlem Globetrotters. This time, there's no possibility of a Vikings win, but the standing-room-only crowd goes wild with the fun.

These activities, plus the usual training room socializing and the drinking scene, keep Karl away from home more and more. I am mainly by myself in the evenings, since he's around maybe only two out of seven evenings. The best description of our life together is mutual love for each other (mostly expressed in bed), mutual love for our son, mutual party going and all the schmoozing necessary for a Vikings player and his wife, but otherwise two ships passing in the night.

As usual, money is tight, and I've found a way to supplement our income. I have, it seems, a very rare blood type that's missing some of the lesser-known antigens and is perfect for the research being carried on in one of the labs. Despite my anemia, I will have one tube of blood a week withdrawn (twelve milliliters, or about a third of an ounce), and I will be paid fifty dollars for it! It isn't enough blood to make any difference with my anemia, so I will keep selling this small amount of blood for several years to add two hundred dollars a month to our bank account.

I've now missed my second period and haven't told Karl yet. Sure enough, I begin to spot again, though there is no pain or cramping like last time. I visit Dr. Stromme, and he tells me that my exam suggests I am indeed pregnant, with a due date of October 1. The pregnancy test is positive, which he says is a good sign. He cautions, however, that only time will tell if I'll miscarry again, and there's not much point going to bed rest to try to prevent a miscarriage. "If you're going to miscarry, you will miscarry, and there's no help for it. You might as well just get on with your life."

The spotting continues, but I don't miscarry. Finally I tell Karl and the world that we're expecting again. He's ecstatic. He runs to phone his parents. "Yep, we're expecting again! Isn't that super?!" He hugs me and lifts me clear off the ground in a wild embrace. He just glows. No one can ever say that he doesn't love his kids.

The off-season continues the same as previous ones, and this pregnancy I am not sick, just bleeding every day during the entire pregnancy. I'm still anemic, so don't feel very strong. And my faithful Irma tells me she will not be able to care for two small children, so I'll need to have another childcare option lined up when the baby is born.

One of my research papers is accepted for a presentation in New York on my due date. I don't worry much about it just yet, as Kurt was born two weeks early, so I assume this little one will arrive early as well. And I'm not nervous about the presentation, because in the last two years I've presented my research at conventions of the Society of Hematology and the American Society of Immunologists in Boston and Philadelphia.

I'm not looking very pregnant yet in April. Senior medical technology students are required to wear a white uniform, basically a nurse's uniform, right down to the white shoes. One day I want to get a clothes item from Schlamps on the way home from school, the same store where I purchased my blue leather coat with the fox collar. But apparently because I have the white uniform on, the salespeople don't recognize me this time.

The main floor sells fur coats and fancy dresses. When I enter, the clerk rushes up to me almost the minute I get in the door and actually takes me by the arm and pushes me toward the elevator. "The sports clothes and other casuals are upstairs," she says. It's very clear she wants me out of the exclusive section in a hurry because I'm wearing a middle-class uniform. She doesn't want her exclusive clients to feel they are shopping in an ordinary store.

I am totally insulted, not that I would be considered unsuitable to be in the expensive clothes section, but that the clerks would treat anyone in this way. I want no part of this kind of snobbery and resolve never to shop there again.

As a young girl (I'm now twenty-two and don't even think of myself as a young girl anymore), I worked for six years in a retail store. Our boss taught us an urban legend and told us to stick with that knowledge, which I always did. Because of his lessons, I usually ended up with big bonuses for my sales acumen, which included treating all customers with respect, no matter what. He said: "There is a legendary luxury department store in Dallas called Nieman Marcus. It's like Saks Fifth Avenue in New York. Maybe even more luxurious. One day, a ragged-looking lady in shorts and a grimy shirt entered the store barefoot. She seemed dirty, smelled of cigarette smoke, and had stringy hair and bitten fingernails. The clerks had all been taught to respect all customers. Their manager told them that looks can be deceiving, so they were helpful and solicitous with this woman. In the end, the woman spent a million dollars."

I remember this story while I am being hustled to the elevator. I don't bother to tell the clerk I've come for a gown for an exclusive country club event. I just turn around and march out the door.

FINALLY, EARLY June rolls around. I'm graduating with a bachelor of science degree in medical technology! I'm also noticeably pregnant. My parents are present from Boone, and Karl is in the audience with them, lovingly holding Kurt and very proud of me. I can see his beaming face in the mass of happy faces.

It's a rainy day, and thousands of students are graduating (there are around sixty thousand students at the University of Minnesota now). The ceremony is held in the football stadium. I'm wearing cap and gown, but the ground is nothing but muck, so I'm barefoot, as are many of my classmates. Under the cap and gown, I'm wearing maternity shorts and shirt.

The program lists my name along with the thousands of others. We are placed by degree and major, and that is how we will walk across the stage—in groups. Mine is listed among several new medical technologists. They'll read our names as we pass with our muddy bare feet (the audience chuckles at the sight of so many dignified students passing the university president with dirty toes sticking out from beneath our gowns), and we're handed a generic diploma. The exact diploma will arrive later in the mail. I'm noted in the program with all the students who have earned a high grade point average. It's a fine day, and I'm so elated and relieved to have made it, despite all my other obligations and complications. It took me five years, but part one is done!

I've made the decision now to try to get into medical school. I don't care what Karl's parents want. This isn't their life to live—it's mine. But it's too late for this year's class, and anyway, I'm having a baby right after the school year starts. So I set my sights on entering the 1968 class at medical school. Of course, it's naive to think I will be accepted. Almost no women are, and I'm not only a woman, but I'm married and will have two children. No matter. I push blissfully forward with my plans and complete my application for the 1968 class. Plus, I have a contingency plan. I'll enter a PhD program in anatomy if I'm not accepted at medical school. The first year of the program is identical to the first year of medical school, and I'll just wait for the usual dropouts from the medical school class, then finesse my way into one of the empty spots. I have no idea if this would work, because I never have to go to this Plan B.

I continue right on working on my research throughout the summer. One day when I'm quite pregnant, one of the PhD research doctors from another laboratory is talking with me when he notices the acrobatics my baby is performing in my tummy. This baby is quite different from Kurt. Unlike Kurt's docile intrauterine stay, this one moves constantly and vigorously, and the punches, kicks, and rolls are quite evident to everyone.

This doctor and his wife have been infertile. They are good friends, and I know of their plight. Right now he's looking longingly and with fascination at my tummy. Suddenly, he asks permission to place his hand on my belly and feel this life growing inside me. Of course I allow it, and he seems transformed. He just keeps his hand still, while the baby obliges him with all sorts of vigorous motion. His eyes tear up, and I am touched.

What he cannot know is how very deeply I am affected by this. Karl hasn't felt this child move or placed his hand on my tummy in any way, let alone with this kind of reverence. I'm nearly in tears too, and I have to turn my head away.

Another vivid scene takes place shortly after this. All of the laboratory personnel chat back and forth. We're one giant family. A while back, someone in the blood bank explained to me that outdated blood for transfusions is great fertilizer for evergreens. Apparently they thrive with the extra iron, and she offered me a supply of this old blood. So all spring I've been bringing outdated blood from the blood bank home and digging it into the earth beneath all the evergreen shrubs and trees I planted around our Burnsville home.

In 2010 this the stuff would be considered a biological hazard and disposed of very carefully. But we aren't afraid of diseases from blood in the sixties. So to keep my evergreens healthy (my editor will laugh at this story and call my trees "vampires"), I occasionally bring home a crate of outdated blood in glass half-liter bottles.

A new freeway, the Crosstown (State Highway 62), is under construction, but there are still some stop-sign intersections, not for the freeway, but for those wanting to get on it. One day I have to take the Crosstown to get to my prenatal appointment with Dr. Stromme. I'm cruising along at fifty-five miles an hour, with a large cardboard box of bottles filled with old blood on the front seat, when the unexpected happens.

A woman pulls up to one of the stop signs and looks straight at me. I can see her blue eyes. She then pulls onto the freeway and stops, cutting off both lanes in front of me. I slam on my brakes but can't avoid hitting her without going in the ditch, which I head for. By some miracle, my car squeezes between two guardrails, missing them by an inch or so, and flips into the ditch, ending up on its nose. I'm hanging up in the air because of the waist seat belt and am not injured, but the bottles of blood were not secured and have smashed all over the windows, bathing them in a sea of crimson.

I see this obviously frightened woman drive on through the intersection and pause long enough to look at my car upended in the ditch, the interior covered in blood. Then she accelerates and is gone. I've often wondered how many hours or days she tortured herself with thoughts of having injured or perhaps killed someone. Did she watch the news to try to find out any information? Did she follow the newspapers? Did she care at all? I'll never know, but I do chuckle at the possibility that she will suffer for not stopping, at least, to help me.

No police ever arrive. This occurred long before cell phones. But soon a kind man with a tow truck comes along, sees my predicament, and easily pulls me out of the ditch. He cleans off the blood on the windshield and will not accept any money for his help. I'm so grateful, I give him one of Karl's autographed photos. I always carry some in the backseat. He's surprised he's helped a celebrity, and I can see that just telling this story over and over to his family and friends will be sufficient payment for him.

Of course, my white uniform is covered in blood, and I create quite a scene when I walk into Dr. Stromme's office for my visit. The receptionist gasps and rushes around the counter to admit me to the exam rooms and table. My blood pressure is very low naturally, which she has forgotten, so she's afraid I've gone into shock from blood loss. I try to reassure her that I am not hurt. Dr. Stromme comes in very quickly, just as rapidly sees I am not hurt, and has a good laugh at this weird story. "I can always count on you to brighten my day, Mrs. Kassulke!" That will be the last time I bring blood home, though.

+∽+

I'T'S NOW a lovely summer, and I'm conspicuously pregnant. We spend another week on Lake Superior with our friends from Duluth. This time we cross the entire lake and go to Houghton-Hancock, Michigan. The lake crossing is rough, a lot like ocean travel, which I discover makes me quite seasick. It isn't the same as travel along the shoreline or between the Apostle Islands. So I spend much of the trip in a bunk, miserable. Karl mostly stays on deck, fishing and drinking with the guys. He isn't especially worried about me.

They don't stick with beer, either. This boat is well stocked with very expensive liquor. They regale each other with stories and jokes, and I can hear sporadic bursts of laughter. I am not feeling very jolly, though. The weather on the open lake is remarkable, with frequent sudden storms appearing and kicking up the waves or distant storms dumping a black curtain of rain while we're still under a blue sky. All of this, however, contributes to my misery.

The canal that winds between Houghton and Hancock is quite charming, with Dutch windmills and beautifully preserved heritage mansions lining its shores. Here the water is calm, and I enjoy the scenery. The area is a copper-mining district, and when we moor for the night, I get off and walk around, picking up several large nuggets of native, pure copper. It's really a quaint area of the country, and I'm grateful for the opportunity to see it. But the trip back across the lake is torturous again, the nausea unrelenting, and I know I will avoid ocean travel or big lake travel in the future.

And then suddenly the guys are gone again to training camp. I'm pretty busy this year with research, Kurt, and finishing all the requirements necessary to apply to medical school. One very hot day, when I'm eight months' pregnant, I take the very important all-day MCAT exam. This examination will be one of the deciding factors of whether I'll be admitted to the medical school class of 1968. My baby is particularly active all day. So the heat, tummy acrobatics, and a backache combine when I'm trying to concentrate on the examination that might mean my entire future. It'll be a month before I know how I did, and it's very tough to wait for the results.

When the letter finally comes, I'm thrilled to see my scores are very high, plenty high enough to be admitted to medical school. But I can't call Karl, as he's at camp, so I just have to wait until his next call. I call my parents instead, and they're so happy for me. I can hear the pleasure and pride in their congratulations. It's two more days before Karl rings me.

"Wow, guess what? I got a great score on the MCAT! I have a chance to get into med school."

"That's great, Janny, if that's what you want. I'll be home in a few days, and you can tell me all about it. I have to get off the phone right now. There's a line of guys waiting."

So I've completed the exam, the application, and the essay, and I have the necessary grade point average. I also have wide cocurricular activities and knowledge with all my music activities. The medical school at this time is very interested in evidence of curiosity and reading and activities in addition to academic achievement. And thanks to my years of working in the medical school research labs, I have some wonderful reference letters. All that remains of the application process will be an appearance before a panel of the medical school doctors. This isn't necessary for all applicants, just special cases—like a married woman with two children. My appearance is scheduled for early October.

Meanwhile, I have to finish preparations for the paper I'll give in New York on October 1. Everything has to be perfect, and I prepare the graphs and other slides that will illustrate my results.

And then there's my baby, also due on October 1. Everything is going to work out, though, because I'm already ripe; the end of my womb (cervix) was widely dilated by September 1. This means the opening to my uterus is thin, soft, and open three centimeters. These findings on my exam suggest imminent delivery, so I'm certain I'll be able to get to New York by October 1.

Karl arrives home from training camp, and Dr. Stromme, Karl, and I all agree to induce the delivery on September 16, two weeks before my due date. Karl, in particular, feels this will be a great day, as the team is playing in town the next day, and he'll be around. By now, my cervix is four centimeters, and Dr. Stromme is actually worried that if I go into labor outside the hospital, I'll have my baby in the car. This is hard for me to imagine, after my last labor.

Karl brings me to the hospital at nine o'clock on the morning of September 16. Dr. Stromme arrives soon after and breaks my water, using a mean-looking metal hook to snag the amniotic sac that is bulging in front of the baby's head, and the water gushes out. He leaves, and I settle down for what I assume will be another long labor time with Karl and all the good feelings when our baby arrives.

Nothing happens at first, except a lot of leakage. After an hour, Karl suddenly stands up and announces he has to leave to make a television commercial. I'm stunned. He hasn't mentioned this before. Why did we schedule this for today if he's busy with something else?

"Don't worry. I'll be back in plenty of time." And out the door he goes without even a kiss good-bye.

Labor sets in about an hour later and is immediately intense. I'm alone and quiet with the pain. I know what to expect this time. One of my med tech friends who now works in the laboratory at Abbot Northwestern Hospital stops by my room. My eyes are covered with a cool cloth, so I don't see her enter.

"Who's making all that racket in here," she loudly barks. I'm being quiet as a mouse and am already mad that Karl is gone. I rip the cloth from my eyes, ready to slug her, when I see who it is. Then I realize it's a joke, and we laugh, both at the joke and my fierce reaction to it.

Things go so fast, I call for the nurse after just an hour of labor and say, "Quick, this baby's coming. Quick! Quick!"

Dr. Stromme makes it just in time to catch little Kory Adam Kassulke, a very different little boy than Kurt. Kory weighs six pounds seven ounces, has very thick black hair—so much hair it covers his forehead and runs down to his shoulders. He has the Kassulke muscular build and normal legs. Later I will see in baby picture comparisons that he has my looks and Karl's coloring, exactly opposite from Kurt. Kory starts out smaller than Kurt and will always grow very nicely in the average range for a man. But he will have the Kassulke muscles and coordination, and like Kurt, he will be a spectacular sportsman, musician, and student.

Kory is whisked off to the nursery, and I return to my postnatal room. I'm alone, without a roommate. Karl doesn't return until evening, and he's drunk. He's surprised to find the delivery over. I guess he's happy to have another son, but there is no warm glow this time, no sense of our working together to get this guy delivered. After two days in the hospital, Karl takes me home, where Kory is installed in his newly prepared nursery. Our house is plenty big enough for both kids to have their own rooms. This turns out to be a good thing, as Kory grows.

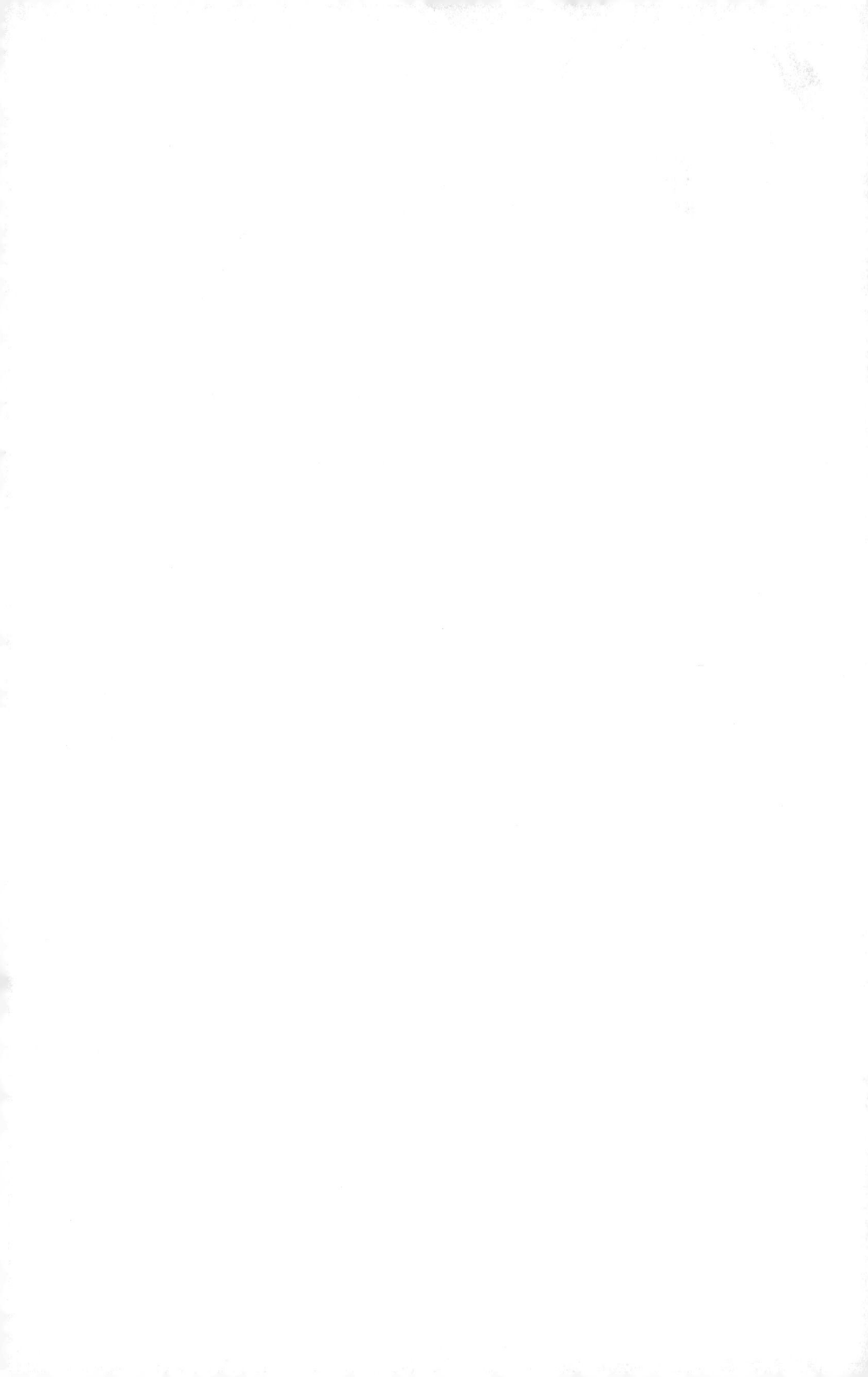

Chapter 14

Surprise!

*T*HE SEASON STARTS AGAIN, and so does the cycle. The promise of a good season is there, especially with an unusually large and talented bunch of rookies, including Alan Page (a thoughtful, studious, future justice of the Minnesota Supreme Court). He completes an already competent defensive line, the other players being Carl Eller, Gary Larsen, and Jim Marshall. As a group they will achieve league fame over the next several years as the Purple People Eaters, due to their near impenetrable line and ferocious tackling. They work together as a smooth machine and are awesome to watch.

The weather changes from mild fall to bitter cold in the stadium. The parking lot tailgate parties, the bridge games, the separations, the groupies, the guys coming out drugged and shower-clean after the game, the postgame parties, the media attention, the tensions, the joys—they all come around again. There are some new faces and some old ones are gone, but basically everything is pretty predictable now regarding the season, except, of course, how many games will be won. This season the expectations are high, but the final win tally is a very disappointing three wins, eight losses, and three ties.

I've been feeling well after this pregnancy and suffered no bleeding disasters. Actually, I'm a little puzzled because I've had absolutely no bleeding after Kory's delivery. Not one drop. That doesn't seem right. Then, one day when Kory's a week old, I start to notice a foul smell in the room. At first I think it's the room, but it turns out the smell travels with me everywhere I go. I can't imagine what's going on until suddenly, the unexpected happens again.

I pass from my vagina a huge wad of extremely foul-smelling gauze. It seems Dr. Stromme has forgotten to remove the packing placed up there while postdelivery repairs were being done. No wonder I didn't bleed. The thing just sat there and rotted until it finally fell out.

I call Dr. Stromme and tell him what's happened. He can't believe he'd commit such a glaring error, so I tell him I'll bottle it and bring it in, which I do. He looks at it through the bottle, then opens the lid. We are both staggered by the putrid smell.

"I'm so sorry. I can't imagine how this happened. But everything looks all right. I rinsed out all the smelly discharge, and there's no sign of infection. Please accept my apologies for this. I'm so very sorry."

Well, I have no plans to sue him or even change doctors. He's the best, and we're friends. It's a great lesson for me though. Even the best doctors make mistakes and must deal with their shame. Doctors are very, very human.

So I have an adorable new baby, and Kurt is now two and a half years old. Parenting has become a priority. Of course I never miss a game either at home or on television, but I'm also busy preparing for my New York presentation. My mom will come up to babysit both kids while I'm gone.

The conference is seven days long, although I'll present my paper on the second day. But I'm also interested in several other papers being presented. Plus, the rest of the time will be spent with sightseeing and Broadway shows, so I'm really excited. I'll be going with Bernice from the lab, who is also presenting a paper. This is a very large conference, almost two thousand attendees. So it's a big deal.

The first of October arrives. I kiss my family good-bye, and in a reverse scene from the usual, Karl drops me off at the airport. I'm exactly two weeks postpartum.

I meet up with Bernice on the plane, and off we go. Upon arrival, we're ferried to a very large luxury hotel, the Americana, and settle into our shared room. This luxury hotel in midtown Manhattan is no longer standing; another more modern hotel has taken its place. The first night, we go to the lounge, where Ella Fitzgerald is performing, and somehow score two seats right up front. It's pure honey watching and hearing this jazz legend so up close, and I'll never forget this magical evening. After the performance, we both get to bed, as I have to present my paper in the morning.

The presentation goes very well, and researchers from all over the world will be exchanging ideas and information with me for the next several years after they've seen this research. It's a very heady time.

Later in the day, Bernice and I are sitting in the hotel lobby after a session when two businessmen sit down and try to hit on us. I'm amused, since I've just had a baby and still am, apparently, attractive enough for these guys to be interested in me. But after a while, I'm bored, and tell Bernice I'm going to bed. "You know, I'm still a bit worn out after having a baby two weeks ago."

I think the two guys are going to have a cow, they almost choke on their drinks. It's hilarious. A great ending to the day. I love to laugh, and this one was great. I go off to bed—alone. Bernice, who's also married, does not come with me.

During the night, I'm awakened with a terrible pain in my right lower abdomen. I've had my appendix removed as a child, so I know it's not appendicitis. And Bernice isn't back yet, though it's three o'clock.

I try to get back to sleep, but the pain worsens by the hour, and I can't walk upright because of it. It isn't a cramping pain, the kind you would get if diarrhea was on the way. It's a steady crushing pain, and I can't imagine what on earth is the problem.

By 5:00 a.m. it's clear something is terribly wrong, and I'm sweating with the pain. The room's turning black. Even though it's very early, I call Dr. Stromme in Minnesota, describe my situation to him, and he says, "Get on the first plane and get home. I'll see you as soon as you get here."

So at 7:00 a.m. I've packed and am just leaving for the airport when Bernice very sheepishly comes in. It's clear she's spent the night with one or both of those men, and she seems embarrassed that I'm finding out. I don't ask her any questions. There's no time to talk, and anyway, I really don't care what she wants to do with her time. It's her business.

I arrive back in Minnesota and take a taxi to Dr. Stromme's office. It's Saturday, but he's agreed to see me. Karl is already sequestered at the Thunderbird Hotel in preparation for the game Sunday afternoon, so he can't pick me up at the airport, and I can't get a message to him after I see Dr. Stromme.

After examining me, Dr. Stromme says, "I don't know how this can be, but there's a large mass in your right pelvis the size of a grapefruit that wasn't there two weeks ago. That's what's hurting. You just about came off the table every time I touched it. I have no idea what it is, but obviously it must come out. I've scheduled your surgery for Monday. In the meantime, here's a prescription for Demerol to help with the pain."

The Demerol controls the pain well, and I'm able to get to the football game the next day, though I wouldn't be able to tell you much about it. I have to admit I'm worried about this sudden development. It's hard to wait on something unknown like the sudden appearance of a large pelvic mass. And Dr. Stromme hinted it might be something very worrisome, like cancer, since it grew so fast.

My mom is going to stay on and help with the kids after my surgery, so I'm covered there. I'm admitted to the hospital after the game on Sunday, and the surgery takes place on Monday morning. Karl is with me before I go into the operating suite, holding my hand. He's not joking today.

The offending mass turns out to be a large cyst (a sack filled with fluid), benign and attached on a long stalk to my right ovary. The pain has occurred because the cyst twisted on its stalk, shutting off the blood supply, and the resulting gangrene was the problem. On the way out of surgery, Dr. Stromme shows Karl the offending blackish purple grapefruit-size mass. Its long stalk is completely black and leathery looking.

The next day is my scheduled appointment with the medical school admissions council. I must not miss this, because to do so would be an immediate strike against me. Dr. Stromme agrees to let me out of the hospital for a few hours.

So with Demerol on board to allow me to move freely with the severe incision pain, I travel to the university by taxi. Karl is off somewhere and not available to take me, and parking a car and walking would be too much for me.

The committee, all male doctors, is sitting around a large oval table reviewing my application, test scores, undergraduate record, and cocurricular activities. I'm expecting academic and educated questions. Instead, the questions are: You know we've never admitted a married woman before, and certainly not one with children. Who's going to clean your house? Who's going to care for your children? How do you expect to be a wife and student both? Who will cook for your husband? The average medical student has to study for six hours a day, in addition to classwork. How do you expect to do that in addition to your wifely duties?

It's a good thing I'm very calm on the Demerol, or I might be tempted to blast these ignorant men for such appalling and irrelevant questions. My record should make it clear I've already dealt successfully with all these issues. But I have to be careful, as this is the only medical school in Minnesota. I've only applied to one school, while most students apply to many. But I don't have the option to move anywhere else, so I have to get accepted here.

Very mildly, I answer, "Have you ever admitted a married man to medical school? With children?" They sheepishly nod that they have. "Did you ask these same questions of them?" They all look at their hands and shake their heads no.

Then I explain to them that I'm very blessed with a photographic memory and do not have to study long hours. I have a very good study system before tests and easily understand the material. I go on to remind them that many of the classes I've already taken were exactly the same as those for freshman medical students, and that medical technologists took them together with medical students. Plus, our grade curve was often higher than that of the medical students.

I finish with the information that I already have a strong medical background, with my premed study of medical technology, and did not have any trouble with those classes, despite my responsibilities. I feel quite confident I can handle the medical school curriculum, and though I'm a successful researcher, I want to be able to help people more fully and directly by being a doctor. This seems to end the conference, and now I must await their decision. I won't know until January if I'm accepted.

So I return to the hospital and gratefully climb back into my waiting bed. It'll be another five days before I'm released to go home. As far as I know, the medical school admissions committee never learned that they were interviewing me directly from my post-op hospital bed.

⁕〜⁕

THE SEASON continues, and I'm fully recovered six weeks after the surgery. Kory's a good baby, very cheerful and funny but quite different from Kurt in his sleep pattern. Kurt still sleeps a lot, a nap both in the morning and afternoon and early to bed at night. Kory, on the other hand, doesn't seem to care much about sleep. He eats well and isn't crabby, but he's awake a lot, doesn't nap, and often coos and rattles his crib toys much of the night.

At first I worry about his strange sleep pattern, but he isn't demanding and seems content to watch his crib mobile and play with his hands. He only cries when it's time to change his diaper. He's also very quickly developed extraordinary muscle control, and by three months he is crawling and satisfying his endless curiosity about the world about him. He's very unhappy if he's stuck in a playpen, though.

I've found a wonderful day care near the university, operated by Rose Embry, so I begin to take both boys there while I work. I'll work the entire year that I sit out between graduation and medical school. This day care is off campus by about a mile, so I can park my car there and walk the rest of the way. Parking has always been a problem, so this is a relief.

Rose is charmed by both of the boys, and they have other kids their age to play with, including another celebrity child. David Soul, who is a folk singer and actor at the Firehouse Theater in Minneapolis, is also doing some small television roles. He will gain wide celebrity in the seventies as Hutch of the hit television series *Starsky and Hutch.* Also, the daughter of my sorority friend from Drake is there each day, so the kids are perfectly happy and never cry when I drop them off.

In the future I'll shake my head at the casual way we handled transportation with children back then. I own a Plymouth Barracuda hatchback, so I fitted out the back with thick padding and carpet and filled the area with plush toys. The kids traveled that way to the university. They would just roll around like bowling balls whenever I had to stop or turn, and they generally squealed with delight each time. Child car seats and seat belts come much later. No one gives a second thought to child safety in cars. We just try to be careful, of course.

In December I begin to experience deep pelvic pain when Karl and I make love, and it throbs for hours after we're finished. I don't understand this. I've been feeling well, and there are no other signs of trouble. But there's clearly something wrong. The pain gets worse each time we connect, which is many times a week, and then I start to have a fever and chills. While all this is escalating, the first real proof of my fears regarding Karl occurs.

We have an unlisted phone number, of course. Otherwise, fans would be calling constantly for Karl. It has proven an impenetrable fortress so far, and we've always received phone calls only from those to whom we provided our number. One night, at three o'clock in the morning, the phone rings, and I answer it. Karl is a very deep sleeper and rarely hears the phone if he's asleep, so I keep it on my side of the bed.

On the line is someone who identifies herself as Debra. She sounds hysterical, weeping and screaming at the same time. I can hardly tell what she's shouting about, but it seems to be something like, "Karl told me he was going to marry me. He's my lover. And now I have gonorrhea, and it's all his fault!"

If there is actually something like my blood running cold, this is it. I'm so shocked, I have to go immediately to the bathroom and vomit.

Karl hasn't even waked. When I can calm down, I begin to think about the last month of fevers and pelvic pain. Right now, it's even painful to sit down. The jarring of movement feels like someone is pounding a meat tenderizer into my pelvis. In my gut I know that Karl has also given me gonorrhea, though I haven't had any discharge to give me a clue about it. He's said nothing about being treated for gonorrhea, though I know he has to have already received treatment. In fact, when I think about it, I realize he's avoided sex with me for the last week, so he probably found out and was treated. He must have been waiting and hoping I didn't get it.

And how the heck did this woman get our unlisted number? I'll never know how she and others did it. Did she go through Karl's wallet and find it there? Did he give it to her for some perverse reason? Maybe he wanted to get caught. I don't know and can't worry much about it right now. Gonorrhea is much more serious to deal with.

The next day, I visit Dr. Stromme. I don't confront Karl about the call, as I've already learned he'll just deny the whole thing and laugh it off. I'm already tired of useless conversations filled with lies.

Dr. Stromme examines me, then asks me to sit up. His usual smile is missing. There's no twinkle in his eyes right now. I already know what he's going to tell me, and I feel completely frozen.

"Jan, you have a serious pelvic inflammatory disease. It's developed since your surgery three months ago. Your pelvis was clean then. Now you have large, tender abscesses in several areas of your pelvis: behind the uterus, in both your fallopian tubes, and possibly even throughout your entire abdomen, because even your liver is tender. I'll need to either hospitalize you for intravenous antibiotics or give you large shots of penicillin twice daily. I'm so sorry, but I think it unlikely you will have any more children." His eyes fill with tears of sympathy.

I tell him about the late-night call. He takes a culture, and, of course, it's gonorrhea. My pain begins to resolve with twice daily penicillin shots, but I will never be without pelvic pain again, neither will I have a normal, pain-free period, nor have pain-free sex until finally I relent at the age of thirty-five and consent to the complete removal of all my female organs. The operation takes several hours because of all the damage and scar tissue, and I need transfusions because of the blood loss during the surgery. I'll need to take estrogen (the female hormone no longer present naturally in my body) for the rest of my life.

A few years later, when I'm in medical school, another Vikings wife comes to me with the same pelvic complaints, and I tell her to get a culture and see a doctor. Sure enough, she also has gonorrhea. I just can't figure why these guys don't at least use a condom. They're not stupid. They're major risk takers, but too often someone else suffers the consequences.

Of course, there are no more pregnancies. So in return for my unending, encouraging support and love and two beautiful sons, Karl has taken my childbearing ability, my youth, my body, and my ability to enjoy sex. I find that though I'll probably always love him, I can't forgive him this time. I know our marriage is over, but I can't bring myself to make a move just yet. All things in good time, I guess. I'm very confused about all of it, and divorce is still a very big no-no in the culture.

Karl knows something is terribly wrong, though, as I make it clear to him I'm getting the penicillin shots and my pelvis is a ruin. I tell him I know he gave me this horrific problem. He doesn't say much but is very contrite and attentive for several months.

Chapter 15

New Beginnings

*T*HOUGH THE TEAM RESULTS were poor for the 1967 season, the public's love for their team does not flag, and the off-season begins just like all the others. Karl is busy with the basketball team, plus he tries another job. He will work off and on at this job for the rest of our marriage. It involves selling packaging to large Minnesota corporations and will also require a lot of travel throughout the state to service his accounts.

One of his largest accounts is Jeno's Pizza, a Minnesota-grown frozen-fast-food industry, and it requires a lot of attention. I never know how much money Karl actually earns at this job, but he does become more proficient at it than his previous work. He has to learn a new language about gauges of plastic wrap, freezer-burn resistance, and strength of cardboard. For a while, I'm hopeful that this work can satisfy him regarding his insatiable need for attention, but it isn't long before I see his heart isn't in it. He begins to miss appointments and expresses resentment when the responsibilities of the work interfere with his drinking and freewheeling.

Meanwhile, the date on which I should receive notification about my admission status to medical school has come and gone. I've not heard either way and don't understand why. Finally, I can't take the suspense any longer, so I call the secretary of the medical school.

"Hi, it's Jan Kassulke. I am a candidate for admission to next year's class. I haven't received any notification yet, and the deadline was three days ago."

"Oh, yes, Jan. I believe you're on the list. You mean you haven't heard?"

"No, I haven't heard a thing, and I'm feeling very discouraged."

"Well, let me check and see what I can find out."

There's a long silence as she sets down the receiver and goes off to check the records. Then, "Well, I'm so sorry to tell you this"—my heart falls into my shoes at these words—"but we made an error somehow, and your records were sitting on top of the filing cabinet, so you didn't get informed. Actually, you were officially admitted just after your interview with the admissions committee."

I'm so relieved, I would hug this lady if I could reach her, but I'm also a bit miffed at being stuck in limbo unnecessarily until past the due date. She continues, "There is some qualification to your admission, so I'll put you through to the dean."

Now what?

The dean comes on the line. "Before you can enter medical school, you have to complete some additional courses. First, you have to take calculus." (Oh no, the dreaded *C* word!)

"Why do I need calculus, Doctor?"

"Well, you need calculus for your biochemistry and physiology courses."

"But I've already had both these courses with the medical students and did just fine without calculus."

"Sorry, but calculus is a prerequisite for medical school. You must complete a course before the start of the school year."

He also tells me that the three semesters of physics I completed were not enough. I had Physics 1, 2, and 3. Premed students took Physics 4, 5, and 6. I bargain with him, and he says, "Okay, if you just take Physics 6 and get an A in the class, that will be enough."

Well, in addition to mathematics, I didn't enjoy physics at all, where I received my lowest grades of any classes in college. Now I'm going to have to take an advanced physics course and get an A as well. I'll just have to do it if I want to be a doctor.

So I set about to complete the requirements. For the calculus, I opt for a mail-order course from the university. The materials arrive, and I start on the first few pages. I realize immediately I've no idea what the book is trying to teach me. I just don't get calculus at all.

I try for a few days but can't finish even the first pages, so I just forget about it and hope they won't notice. I never complete the calculus and never mention it at the medical school. In the back of my mind, I imagine that at graduation, they will call me on the stage and say, "Too bad, you don't get to graduate because you didn't do the calculus before you entered school." As it happens, something quite different happens at graduation.

For the physics, I enroll in summer school for Physics 6. It turns out to be all the new physics: Einstein's theories, time bending in space, sub-atomic particles, black holes, and other totally intriguing topics. I find I very much like this physics. The tests do require calculus, but somehow I can figure out the answers without knowing the calculus, and I end up with the required A. So I finish the summer before starting medical school, batting 50 percent on the requirements they gave me. Actually, it appears they never even checked to see if I completed anything at all.

My research work has continued, as it will throughout my medical school years. But things are getting sour in the lab. It seems Bernice has fixated on me in a paranoid way. I don't understand why. I've never done anything to cause her trouble, but she begins to loudly complain about me to the higher-ups. They call me in, and it's clear they understand she is being neurotic (at best) for some reason. But the problem goes way beyond neurosis.

She's truly obsessed with me. She announces that she's applying for medical school, and she will also have a second child. She's trying to copy my life. She does actually get pregnant and then miscarries. Then she announces that I caused her miscarriage. How I managed this is never clear to anyone.

She doesn't get accepted to medical school because her psychological examination is suspect. She blames me for this too. It's clear there is serious trouble here, but for some reason no one seems able to do anything about it or takes it seriously. I naively assume all of this is because I know what she did in New York, and she's acting out of guilt. But I've never mentioned any part of her infidelity to anyone.

I truly don't understand the depth of her mental illness until I arrive at work one day to find a curious problem, which takes me a moment to figure out. My desk is under a reverse flow hood, due to the radioactive tritium bottle there. The air is sucked away from the lab and me by this hood, which safely removes all radioactivity out of the area. This day I notice my desktop is sticky. At first I get a cloth to clean it, then I stop to think what might be so sticky. On a hunch, I check the tritium bottle and discover it's empty. Completely empty.

I have to account for every milliliter of this radioactive liquid in a logbook, so I know I left this bottle nearly full yesterday. Someone has spilled the entire bottle on my desk and let it dry down. We get a Geiger counter, and sure enough, my desk is highly radioactive.

I don't know if working at this desk for long would actually have killed me or made me sick, but someone evidently thought so. I'm sure I know who that someone is. Bernice is removed from her job in the lab and spends time in a psychiatric hospital as a full-blown paranoid schizophrenic.

⁺〜⁺

BUT FOR now, it's a fine summer before I start medical school. Karl and I take our usual Lake Superior summer cruise with our Duluth friends. It's gorgeous, as always, along this truly spectacular body of water. The water is clear and cold, the weather eerie and unique, the shoreline a constantly moving portrait of natural glory. We don't cross the lake this year, so I'm not seasick and can enjoy everything.

We're thrilled to see eagles, a glorious bird making a comeback from near extinction. We also glimpse deer, moose, wolves, and every manner of water bird as we travel along. The men enjoy themselves with fishing and beer, and I pass my time reading on the front deck and enjoying the view. I'm definitely not spending as much affectionate time with Karl now, though we'll still hold hands when we go places. I've had to cut way down on our lovemaking, partly because I am turned off and partly because it hurts.

The media continue to adore us as a couple, even more now that I'm going to attend medical school. This is a complete novelty in the pro football arena. Though I don't exactly tell the whole truth in interviews when asked about our life together, because I know in my heart that we will not be married forever, I don't lie either. I do truly care for this flawed man. I can even understand some of the sources behind his behavior, but I know I don't want it in my life, and when the time is right, I'll jump ship. I don't make a move now because I don't want to upset Karl and cause him not to play at his best.

I know it isn't about finding the funds to go to medical school. At this time, it costs $250 a quarter, plus textbooks, to go to medical school, and I earn a great deal more than that with my job. Mostly, I want to protect Karl and his career, still being codependent to the very end.

Karl and I also take a great trip to Boone. My mom fixes fabulous picnics with her famous fried chicken. We eat outdoors in the backyard under the giant willow tree. The weather is balmy, with a sweet breeze wafting a newly-mown-grass-and-black-dirt smell. I have a new eight-millimeter camera, so I take film of the picnic, with Karl, Kurt, Dad, and Mom sitting at the picnic table and Kory in his high chair. In later years, Dmitri will digitize these films, and I will watch this idyllic family scene again and send it to my grown-up boys. Karl looks happy, as do my parents, and the boys are really enjoying themselves. I'm not in the scene because I'm behind the camera.

My parents have no idea our marriage is in any trouble. Like most couples at this time, we keep our problems to ourselves.

The team in general has become wilder in their private lives. There are many rumors about bad behavior, and divorce and even suicide among the wives has occurred. By the time I am divorced, there will have been one suicide, perhaps two, and one questionable drowning among the wives. A bit later there will be an early death from anorexia.

It's a risky and challenging business being married to a celebrity. The mortality rate is much higher than in the general population.

Drugs have become a much bigger player. Now marijuana is in general usage, especially on the defensive team, and cocaine, heroin, and a whole group of hallucinogens are now available. Karl dives into whatever's offered him. When he comes home now, he's often not only drunk but also hallucinating and vomiting, and I have to ask him what he took.

"I don't know," he'd answer. "It was a pink and white pill. I took three of them." As he hugs the toilet, he says, "Janny, can you get these bugs off me? Get them off! Help... Help... Get them off! They're going in my nose! No, wait, they're butterflies... Wow! What colors! Oh, there's a blue and purple one on your nose. Careful, don't knock it off."

This would go on for hours, sometimes all night. Then I would call poison control to find out what the pink and white pills are. They always know and give me advice on caring for Karl until he comes out of it. Apparently Karl revels in trying everything, and it's a challenge to keep up with his drug use. So now he's not only an alcoholic, he seems to be into drug use. And he keeps right on driving through all of it.

When we have parties, whether with the team or with other friends, there's now usually marijuana in small quantities. I will enjoy smoking marijuana, but that's as far as my experimenting will go. It's hard for me to smoke because I've never smoked cigarettes, and when I do, I cough and hack until I vomit. It's quite an unpleasant price to pay for the pleasure of marijuana, so I don't do it very often. And I will never try LSD, although most of my friends and the team do. Probably over the next four years, I'll smoke ten joints. I'll have great fun with them, laughing endlessly, traveling in my mind with the increasingly acid-rock music, and feeling great wonder at such things as bread rising in the oven while baking. But when I graduate from medical school, I'll distance myself completely from marijuana because it's illegal at this time, and I'm a doctor. I don't wish to get in trouble (although around 75 percent of the medical students use marijuana).

One event illustrates the state of things at this time. The men are at training camp, and I am visiting in the home of another defensive back. His wife and I are chatting while our kids, about the same age, are playing. She tells me some gossip about one of the defensive players.

It seems the wife of one player in this elite group is having an affair and is currently off camping with her lover, having left her child with a baby-sitter. I'm very surprised. This player is very kind and impressive, and I can't imagine anyone cheating on him. He's probably the straightest and most honest player on the team, but his wife is definitely cheating.

Just then the doorbell rings, and this player is standing on the doorstep. He's been suspicious of his wife and has been unable to reach her (there are no cell phones yet). Even though it's not a day off at training camp in Mankato, he's driven home to confront his suspicions. Sure enough, he finds the baby-sitter at home and no wife. He comes to the home of his wife's friend, knowing she will reveal what is going on.

He's told what's happening and where to find his wife. He goes to the campsite and catches her in the act of infidelity. That's the end of that marriage. I am glad for him when he later marries a woman who appears to be his helpmate, counselor, and soul mate.

I have no time for thinking about an affair, though it does appear I have an open marriage, something that was never discussed with me but is a current fad in the culture. Supposedly, this means both partners continue to love each other but have sex with whomever they wish, whenever they wish, with (supposedly) no risk to the marriage. This is sure not something I ever agreed to.

＋〜＋

KURT AND Kory are now three years and nine months old. Kory has been quite a handful, and things reached a peak this spring when he was six months old. He's cheerful, charming, funny, inquisitive, and unusually well coordinated. But this creates very unique problems. First, he learns by five months to pull himself into a standing position in his crib. He's in the same room Kurt had as a baby, and I haven't changed it much, including the wall of glass-framed clown images that surround the crib nook about a foot above the crib. There are six of them.

One day I come into his room after nap time. He never sleeps during this time but is content to play with a variety of soft toys in his crib. Not today, though. I find him sitting in a large pile of broken glass, playing with the shards. There's not a single scratch on him.

He's figured out how to climb up on the vertical slats of the crib and reach the pictures. Once he had them all in the crib, he gleefully discovered he could bang them together and smash the glass. There's not one unbroken picture. How he managed to avoid serious cuts, I'll never know, but I've learned a valuable lesson: never have any sharp edges or glass where Kory can reach them.

But Kory is always ahead of my prevention tactics. He's learned from this event that he can also lower himself out of his crib. Then he navigates the stairway by straightening his body into a board and just sliding down. He's far ahead of Kurt's activities at this age, and I'm kept constantly thinking how to prevent injury.

Then something far worse happens. One night I am awakened at 2:00 a.m. by the sound of breaking glass. At first I fear someone has broken into the house, so I shake Karl awake. We notice Kory is out of his room, and I feel dread at what we'll find. Our house has three levels, so there are two staircases, all covered with carpet. Kory isn't upstairs in his room, so we search the next level: the kitchen, the living room, and the dining room. He's not there, and we can still hear the noise coming from downstairs.

The next level down is the large family room, thickly carpeted (deep purple shag carpet, of course), and it includes a bar with a large liquor cabinet filled with all kinds of hard liquor. Above the bar is a lighted Hamm's Beer sign with the bear and fish and apparently moving water, the standard fixture in every well-equipped bar of the time.

There's also a closed door that leads to a fourth level, a finished basement. Because the door is closed, we know Kory isn't in the basement (he can't reach door handles yet).

This just leaves the area behind the bar, where we not only hear the breaking glass but can also smell the alcohol. When we reach Kory, he's smashing bottles together, laughing joyfully when the glass shatters and the liquid splashes out and soaks him. Just like before, he's sitting in a huge pile of glass shards and jagged bottles. Just as we arrive, he's finished off the last bottle, and the entire liquor supply is destroyed, which I am not grieving about. He's not injured in any way, not a single scratch.

For a moment I think of the irony that Kory and all this liquor are actually sitting on the purple shag rug that exactly covers the huge blood spot I left on the floor a few years earlier.

Anyway, I quickly pick him up, but Karl reaches for him. "Hey, little buddy. It's kind of early for you to be hitting the sauce like this, don't you think? Honk, honk!" He hands Kory back to me, and I go upstairs to bathe him, because he reeks. As soon as I put him back in the crib, he's quickly back on the floor, crawling off to his next adventure.

So, in the middle of the night, I make a decision that will keep Kory safe, though I probably would be called out for child abuse today. I take his dresser, change table, and crib out of the room and leave the mattress and many blankets on the floor. I remove all other hard objects and toys from the room and fill it with soft toys. I make sure he's warmly dressed in his sleeper pajamas that cover every inch of his body except his head and hands. Then I put him in bed on the mattress, leave the room, and lock the door from the outside.

He's indignant at first and cries and slams against the door, but I will not let him out. Soon he accepts his situation and falls asleep by the door. Until he's well over two years old, he'll sleep in this room each night with the door locked. This arrangement works well, and every morning he's asleep by the door. He has no further harrowing events, and when he's two years old, we give him a toddler bed and furnished room again. He seems to have stopped his nocturnal destructive activities, so we leave the door unlocked, and all is well.

This busy little boy is walking by seven months and a climbing, running, sliding, gleeful little monkey all of his young years. He loves to be read to and adores music as well, but academics will not be his favorite activity—that much is clear. *Activity* is the operative word here. Kory is a busy, active boy and must be watched as much as possible to keep him out of harm's way. I discuss all this with Karl's mom, and she tells me Karl was just like this when he was a baby.

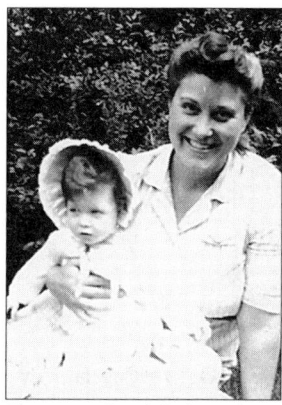 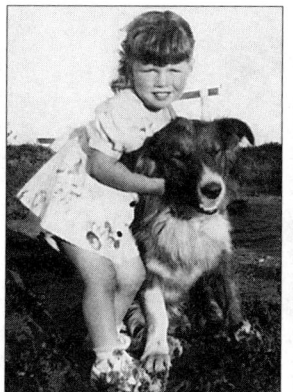 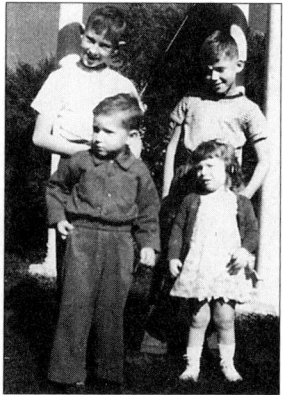

Above, my South Dakota days with my mother, my grandma's farm dog Sport, and my three brothers (clockwise from bottom left) Jerry, Alan, and Bruce.

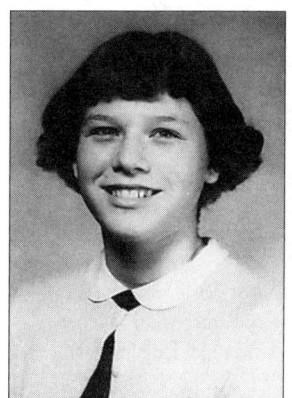 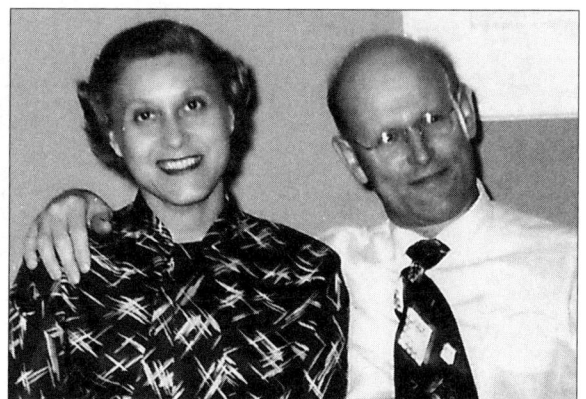

Above are photos of me in fifth grade and my mom and dad, Mildred and Howard Thatcher. Below left, from left to right, I pose with Barb Holscher (the winner) and Patti Whalen in my only beauty contest photo, for D Club Sweetheart. Below right, Karl and I pose at a campus Christmas dance.

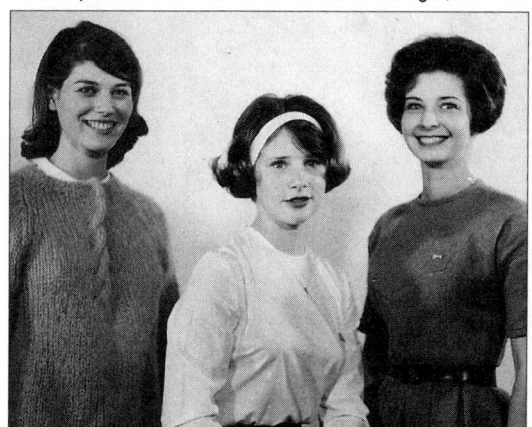 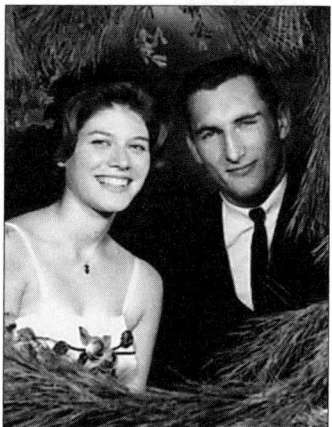

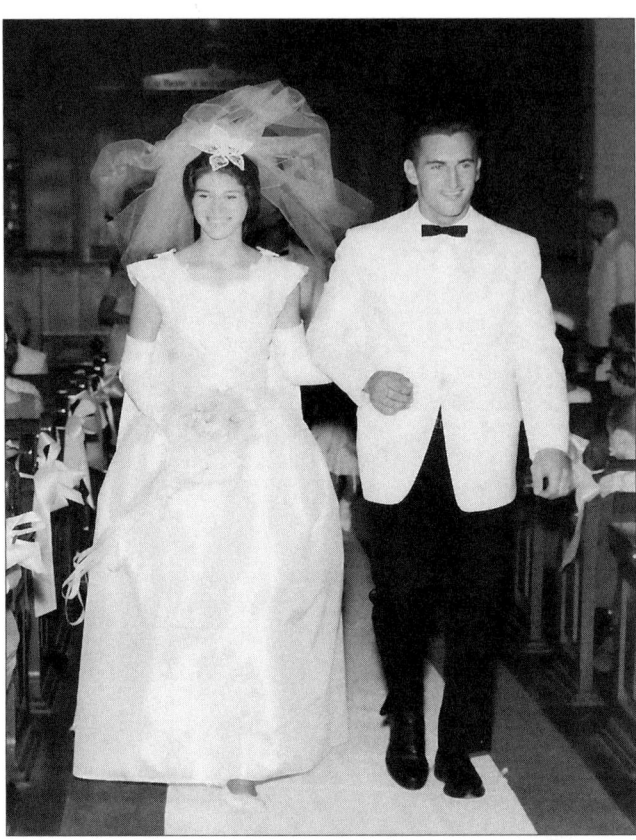

Our wedding day, July 7, 1963, was in the midst of a scorching Iowa summer. And yet it was a fairy-tale event. We had a beefy lineup at the altar, as the five best men were all Drake football players. We were married at the First Methodist Church in Boone, with Karl's brother, Reverend Willard Kassulke, co-officiating with my Methodist minister.

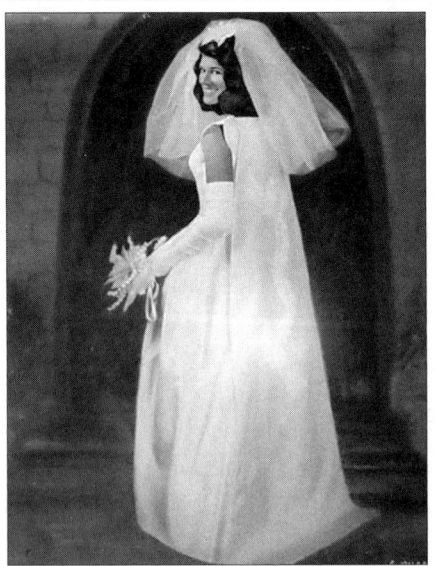

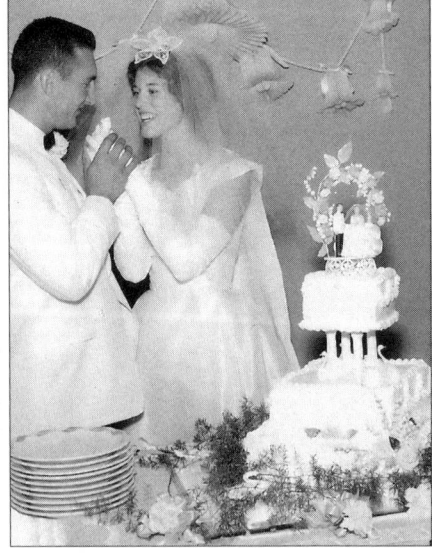

In 1964 I visited my parents in Boone. I am holding Plato and standing beside our new car, which has some visible black angus crunch on the front end. Karl has gone off to training camp in Bemidji, Minnesota.

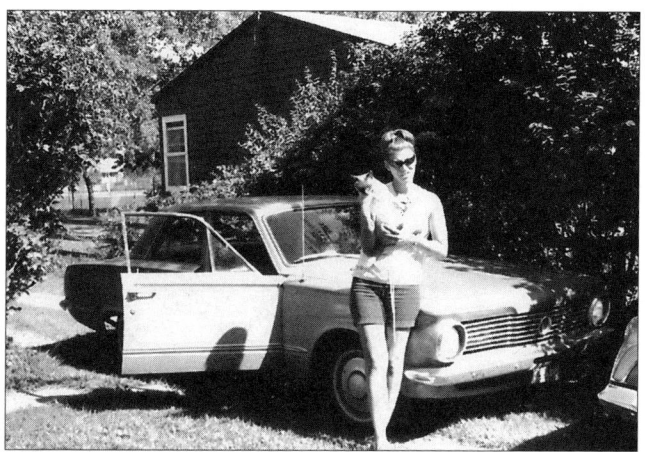

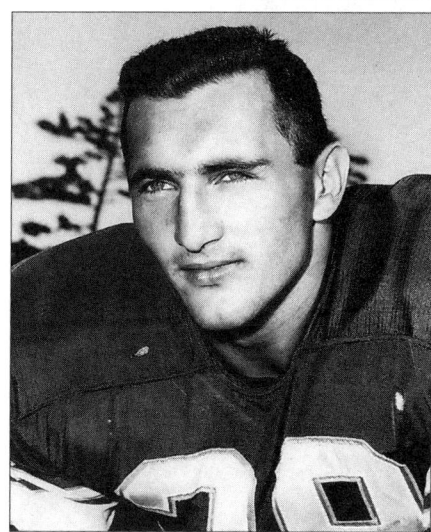

After a disastrous rookie experience in 1963 with the Detroit Lions, Karl was picked up during the preseason by the fledgling Minnesota Vikings. This is a promotional photo of their new, handsome strong-side safety who wore number 29.

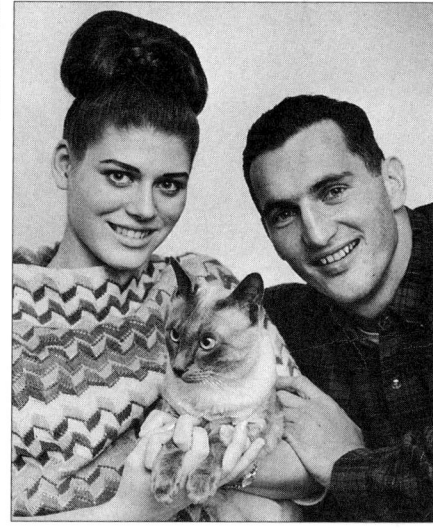

In the fall of 1964, we posed with Mrs. Plato at our Bloomington apartment.

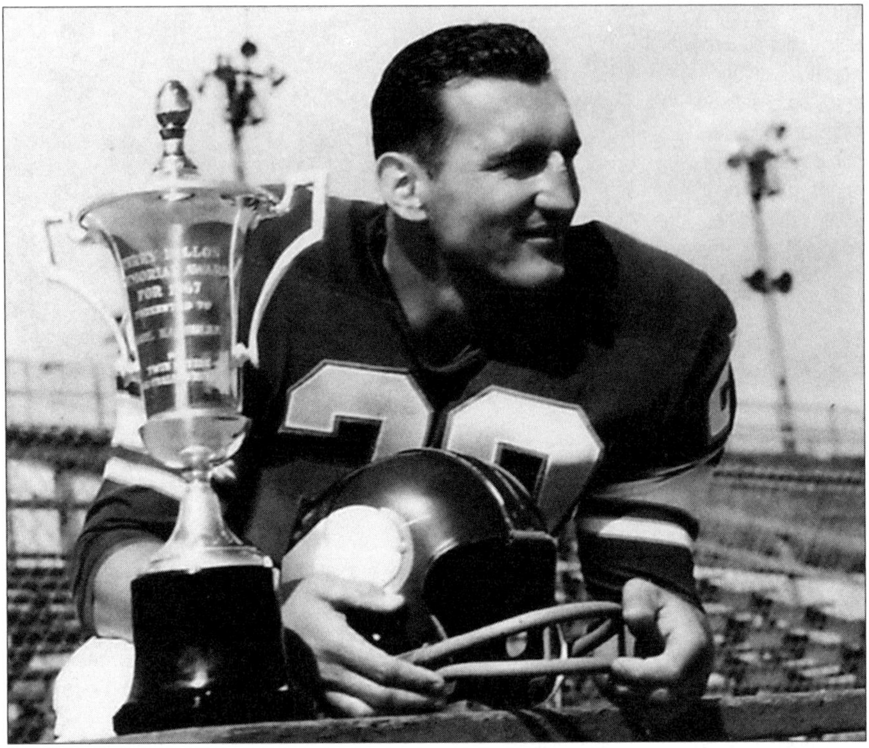

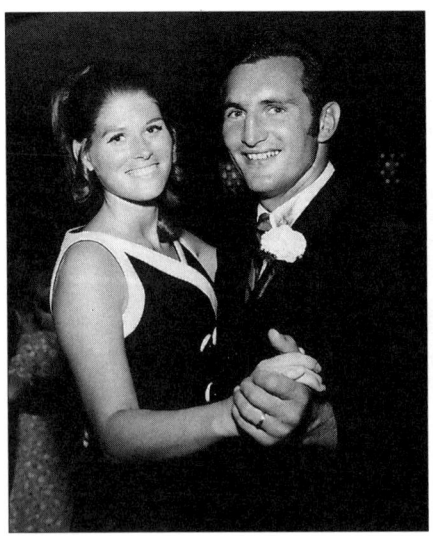

Above, a rightfully proud Karl was honored in 1967 with the coveted Terry Dillon Award. Below left, we loved to dance. Karl taught me to do a rowdy Milwaukee polka. Below right, I took in a show in Las Vegas while Karl stayed at the gambling tables that particular evening.

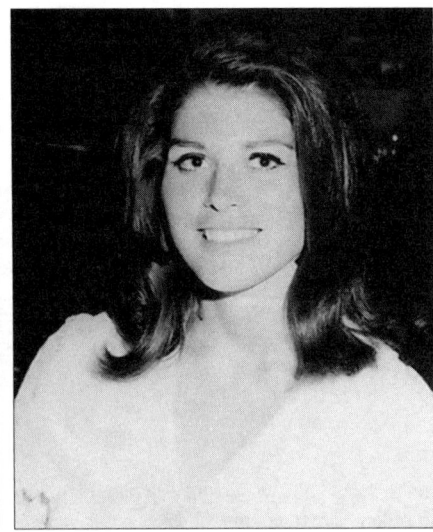

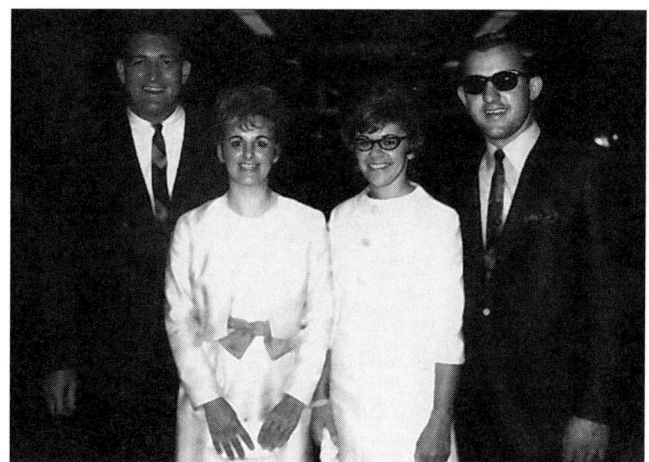

These are some of our Minnesota Vikings friends. At the top, on vacation with us in Hawaii, from left to right, are offensive lineman Grady Alderman, Elaine Tarkenton, Nancy Alderman, and quarterback Francis Tarkenton.

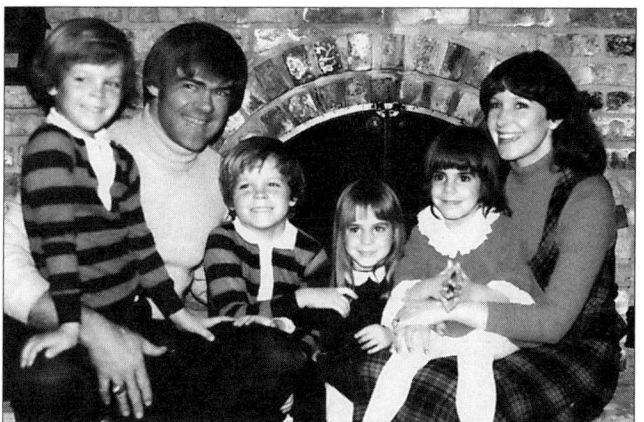

Above are linebacker John and Sue Campbell, with twins Andy and Matt and twins Molly and Meghan at home in Burnsville, beside their fireplace. Below are Marcia and quarterback Joe Kapp and son.

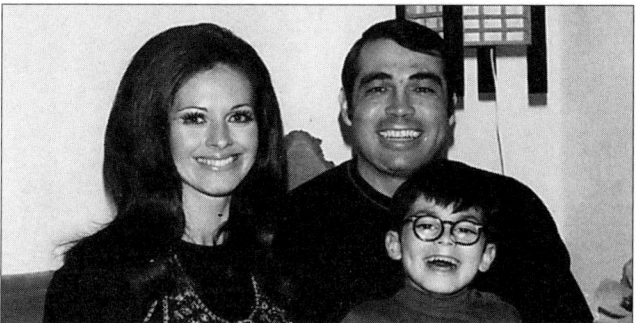

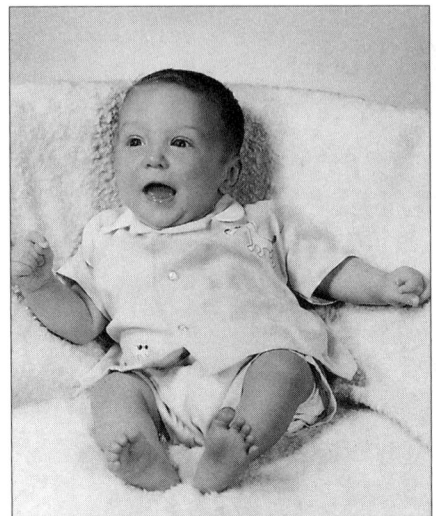
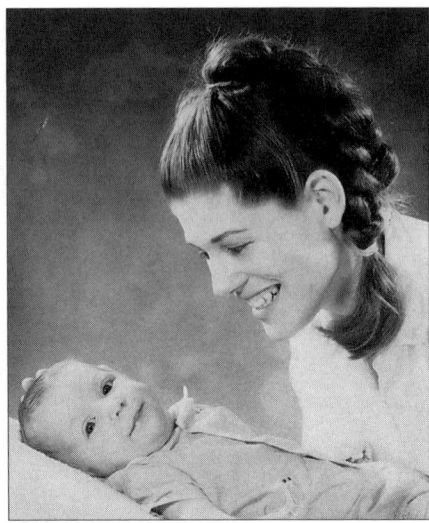

Kurt Alan Kassulke is born in 1965. He is a vigorous baby, but he had two club feet. He underwent a painful series of casts and corrective shoes. When finished, he had beautiful, straight feet and legs. Above left, Kurt is out of his leg casts for a break. A sore big toe didn't phase his sunny personality. Above right, the camera caught me absolutely adoring this little man.

Below left, Grandma Thatcher is getting acquainted with Kurt in Boone. Below right, also in Boone, Grandpa Thatcher holds his latest grandchild. Kurt has a corrective shoe on his right foot.

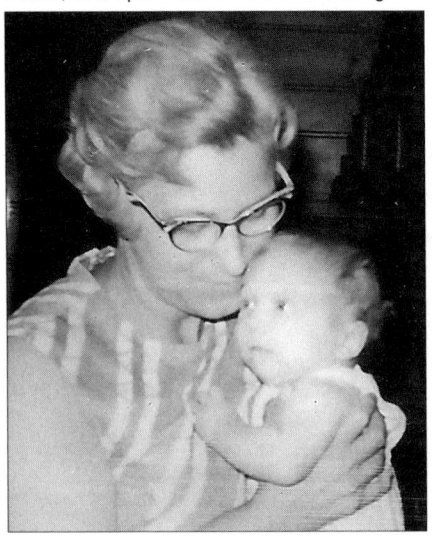
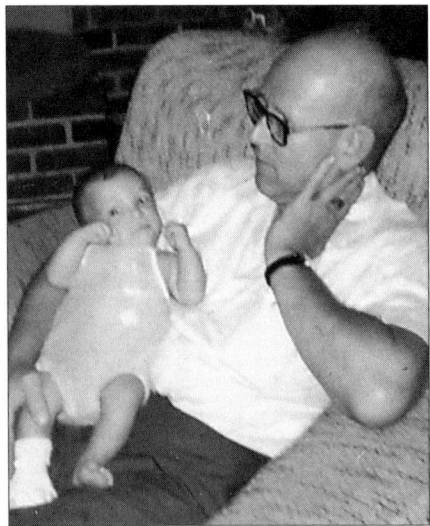

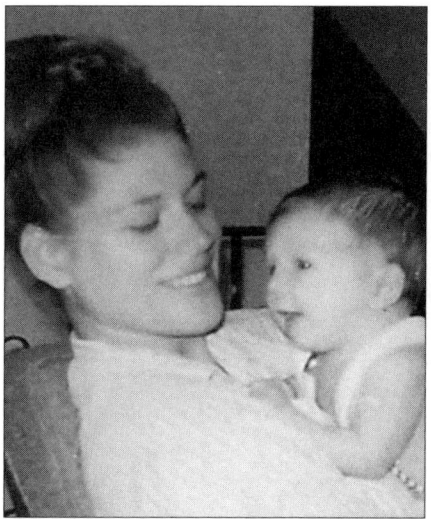 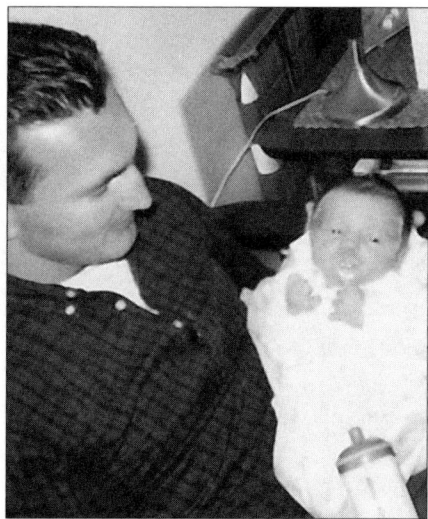

More precious time is captured on film with Kurt. Above left, I am enjoying Kurt's giggle at home in Burnsville. Above right, Karl discovers the meaning of "spit up." Baby photos of Karl and Kurt are nearly identical, except Kurt has reddish blond hair, compared to Karl's dark hair.

Below left, Aunt Christy Kassulke snuggles with Kurt, who is still wearing his corrective shoes. Below right, Kurt can't wait to start splashing and rubber ducking in the tub.

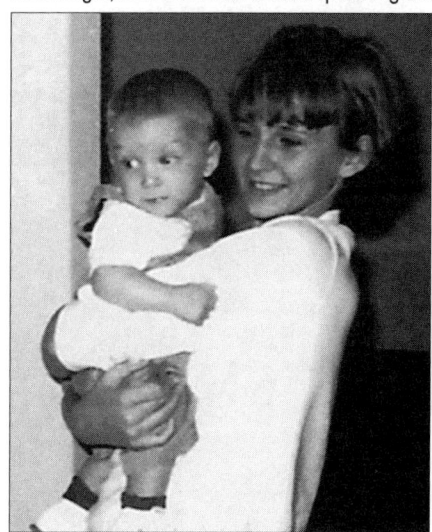 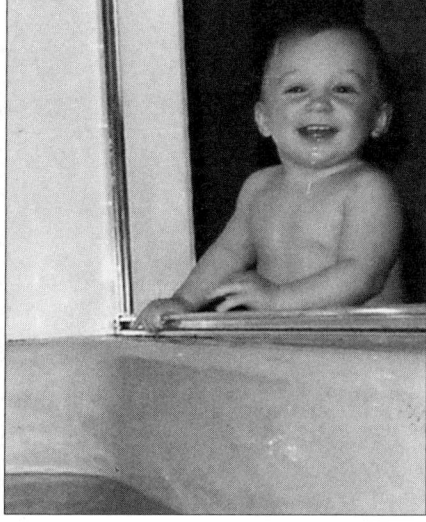

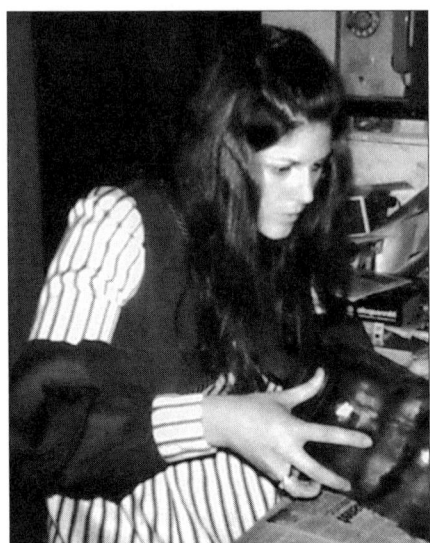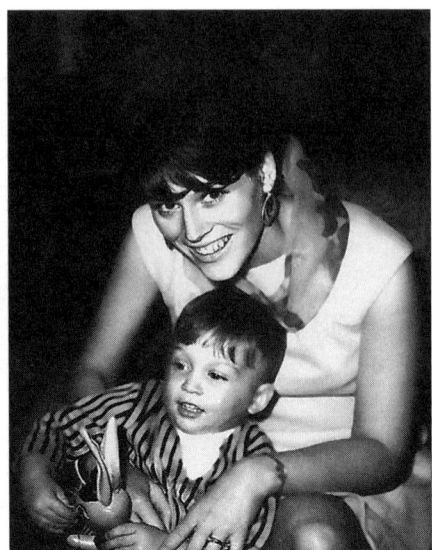

Above left, since I am often home alone, I keep busy with mothering, school, craft projects, and cooking. Above right, I pose with Kurt on an Easter morning in Boone. Kurt plays with the head of his Easter bunny. Below, I am photographed during a performance. I played cello in my high school orchestra, the Des Moines Symphony, the University of Minnesota Orchestra, and the Bloomington Symphony and made various other solo appearances.

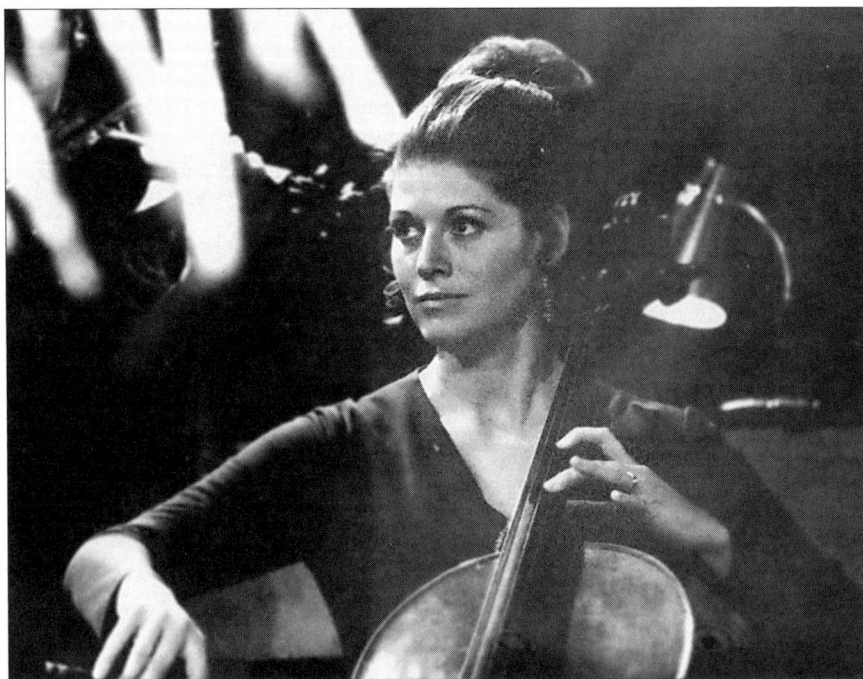

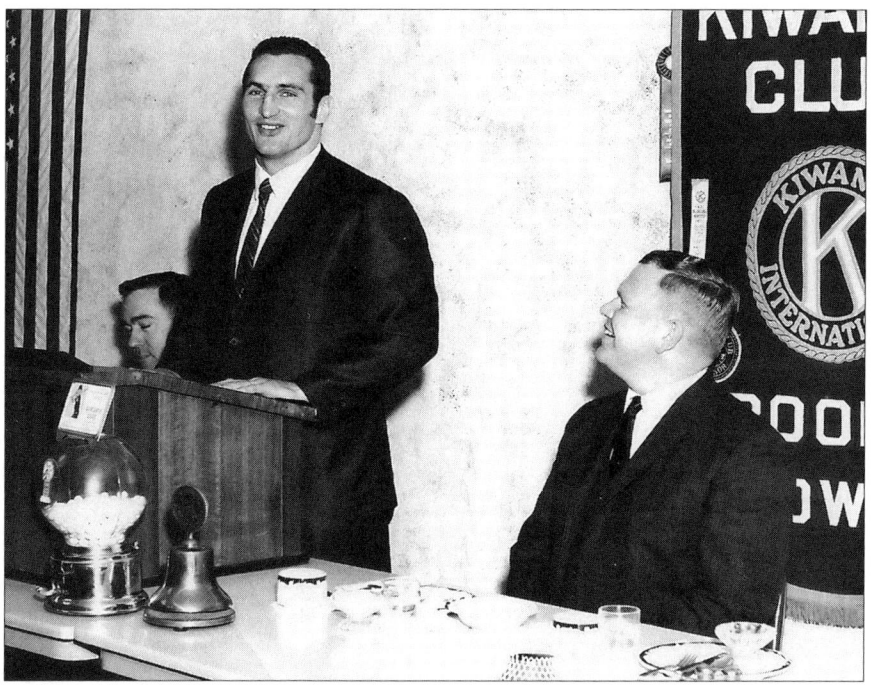

Above, Karl is well received by the Kiwanis Club in Boone, Iowa. He enjoyed public speaking and was very busy with engagements. But while other players earned handsome fees for their public appearances, Karl rarely charged anything, because these events nourished his need for public adoration. Below, we were dazzled by the lush conservatory gardens at Como Park in St. Paul. These photos were taken just before the infamous "panther incident" described in chapter 8.

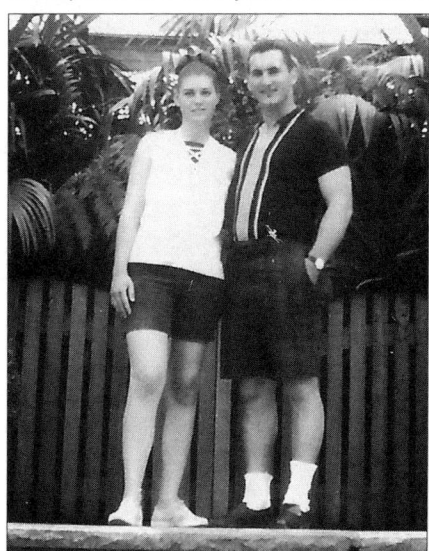
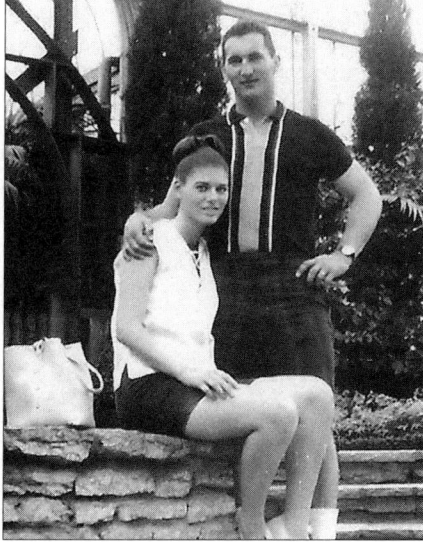

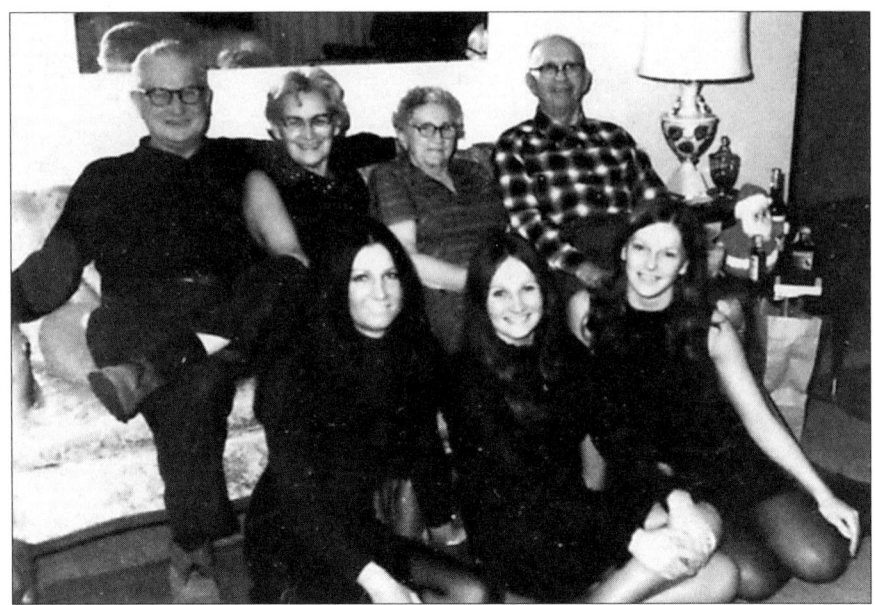

Above, Karl's Milwaukee family (clockwise from back row left), dad Otto Kassulke, mom Leona Kassulke, maternal grandparents the Freitags, and sisters Kathy, Christy, and Carmen.

Below left, Kory Adam Kassulke arrives in 1967. He has Karl's dark hair and complexion but otherwise looks like my baby photos. Grandma and Grandpa Kassulke smile at this little wiggler. Below right, Grandma Kassulke in Burnsville with a growing Kurt.

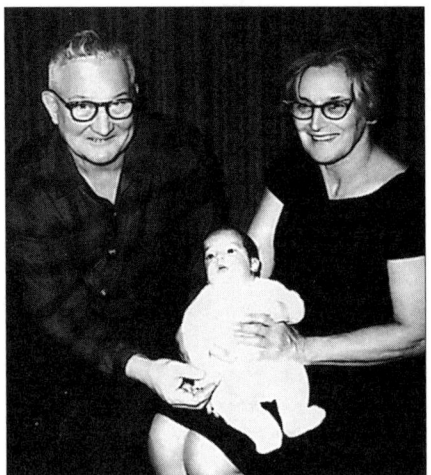
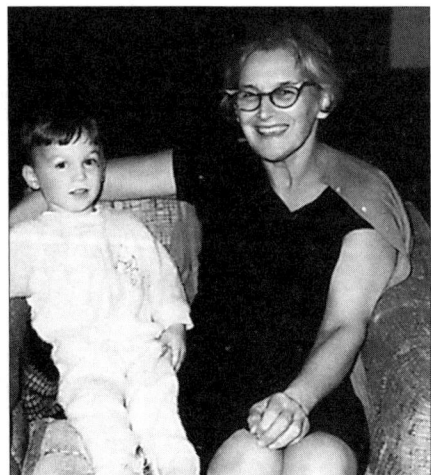

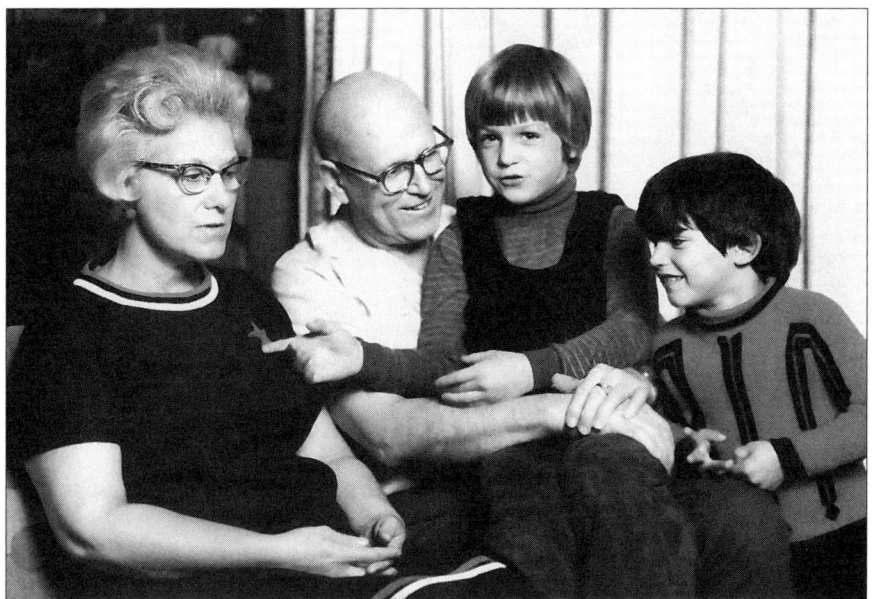

Above, Grandma and Grandpa Thatcher pose in Boone with their inquisitive and cheerful grandsons, Kurt and Kory.

Below left, Grandpa Thatcher, Kory, and Kurt watch television in Boone. Below right, Grandpa Thatcher and Kory in Burnsville smile for the camera.

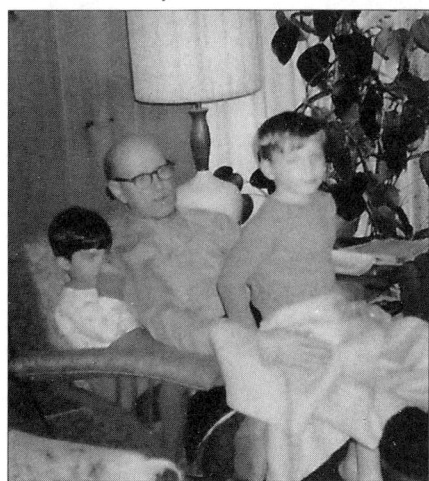

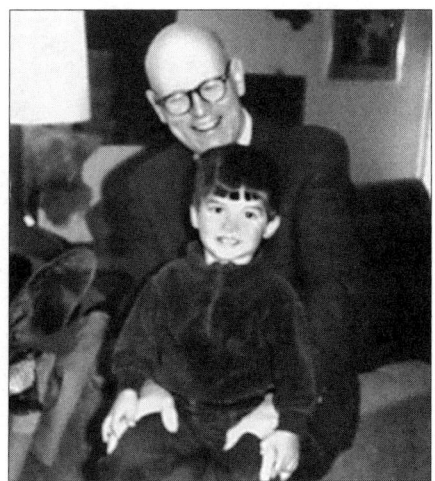

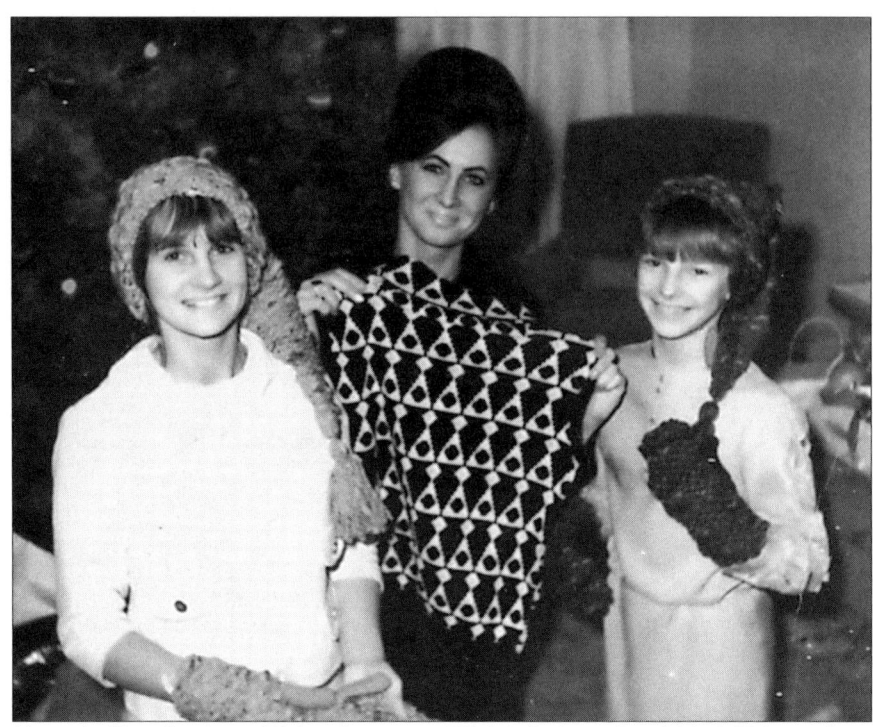

Above, the Kassulke sisters (Christy, Carmen, and Kathy) display and model their Christmas loot.

Below left, I am with Karl's brother, Rev. Willard Kassulke, and his family, Carolyn and Westley. This photo was taken shortly after I chopped off all my long hair. Below right, Willard and Carolyn's family grows as little Dori joins brother Westley.

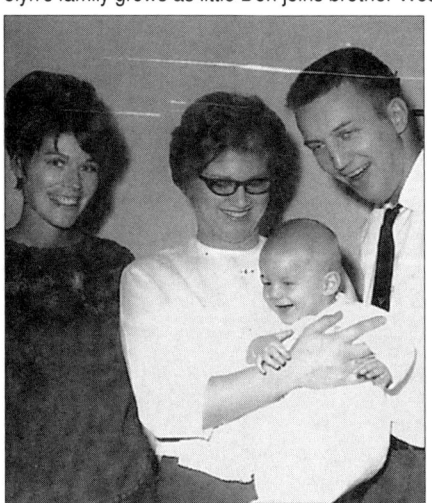

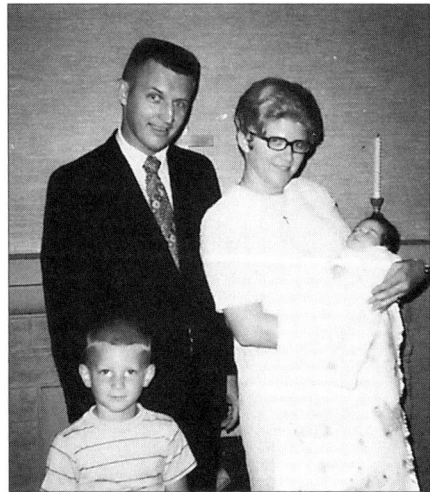

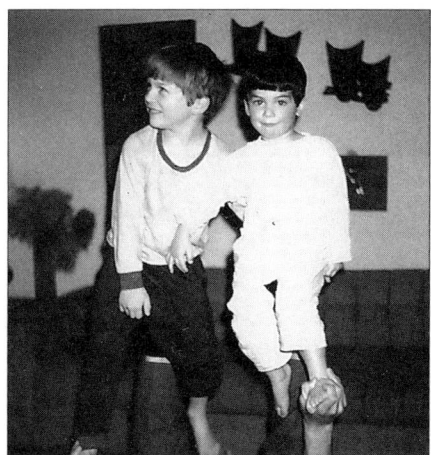

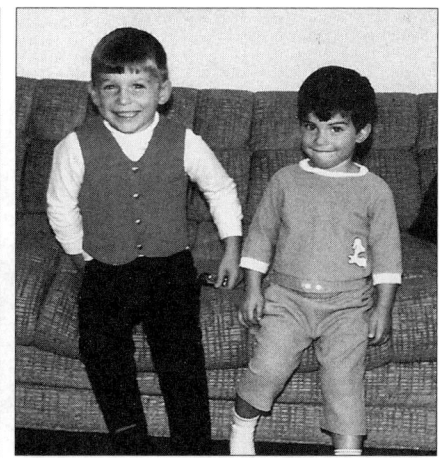

Above left, strong daddy Karl hoists Kurt and Kory during some of playtime. Above right, Kurt and Kory pose all dressed up on the Burnsville sofa. Right, Kory loved to snuggle with his sheepskin. The same sheepskin is still a favorite, forty-one years later, with my cats. Below left, Kurt models an expensive snowsuit at Dayton's Department Store in Minneapolis. Below right, Casey Jones, a local television star, poses with some of the models from the Dayton's show. Kurt is front and center. Casey was one of the moderators of the show. Kurt wore his wonderful snowsuit for one season. Of course, by the next year, he had grown completely out of it.

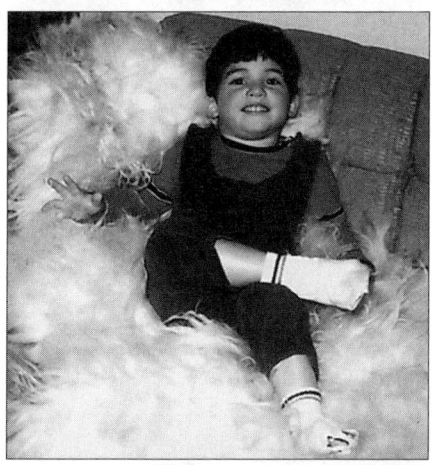

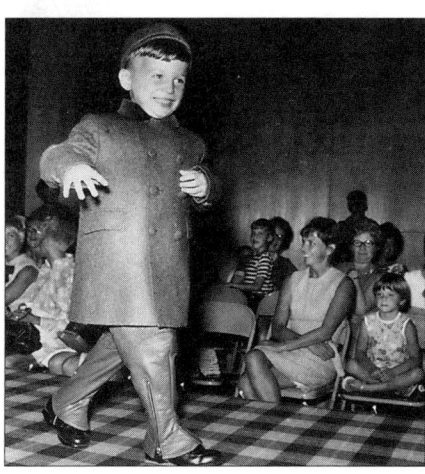

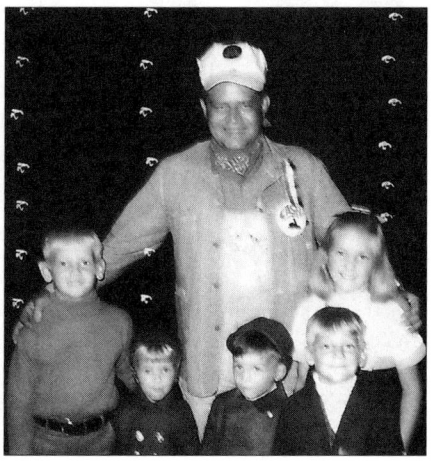

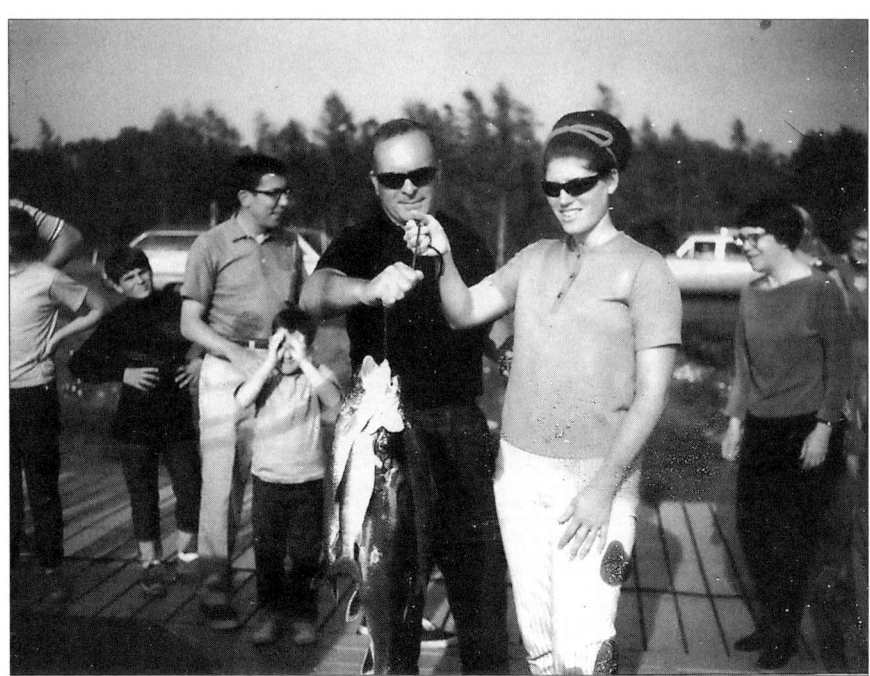

We were all avid fishermen. Above, I'm holding my day's catch of brown trout and Coho salmon from one of our Lake Superior trips. The fish are so heavy that I need help from a friend to lift them. Below left, a happy Karl displays his catch from a day's fishing at a local lake with a buddy. Below right, I have another successful day at Lake Superior. This particular catch was during a time when Lamprey infested Lake Superior, and many of the fish had eels attached to them. It was a fascinating oddity.

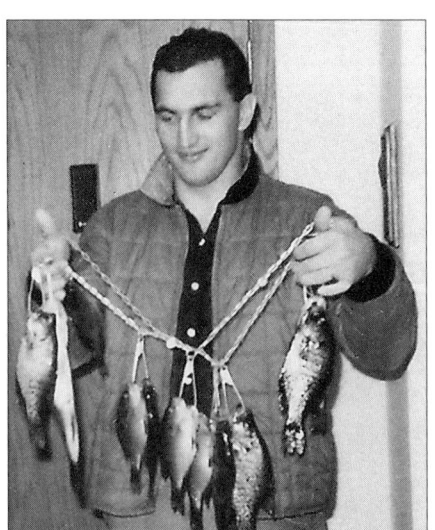

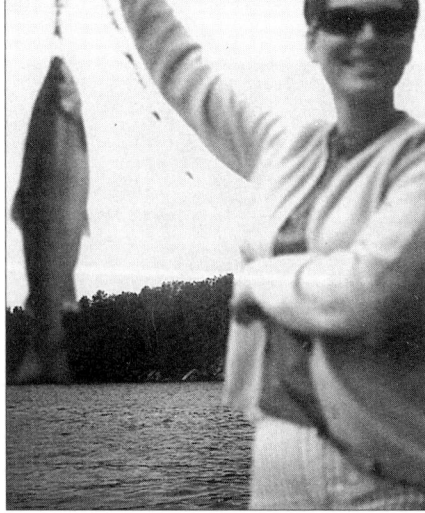

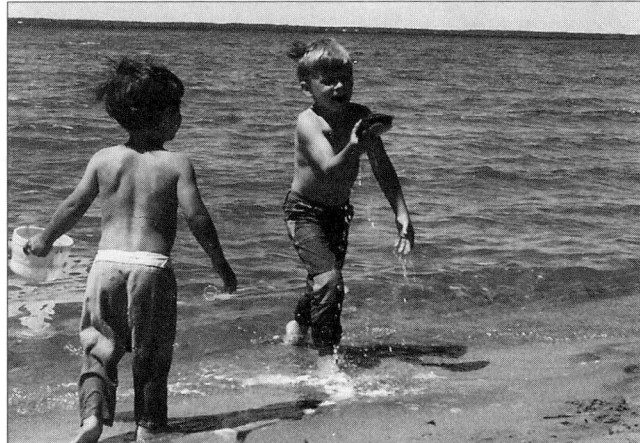

We are at a friend's cabin for our only vacation "up north." Kurt is thrilled with a small turtle, and Kory is wearing long pants to stave off the leeches.

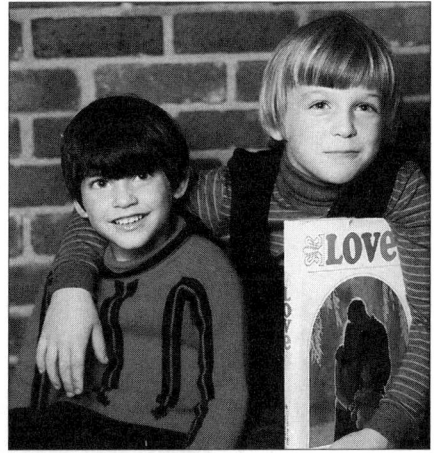

Kurt and Kory pose for Boone neighbors and professional photographers Frank and Juanita Welch.

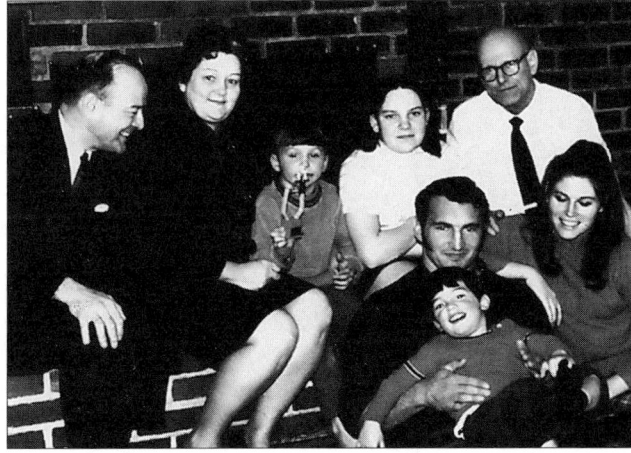

Karl, Kurt, Kory, me, and my dad are in Boone with family friends, the LaMottes.

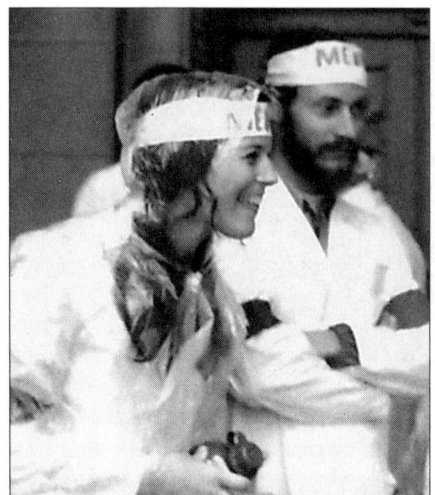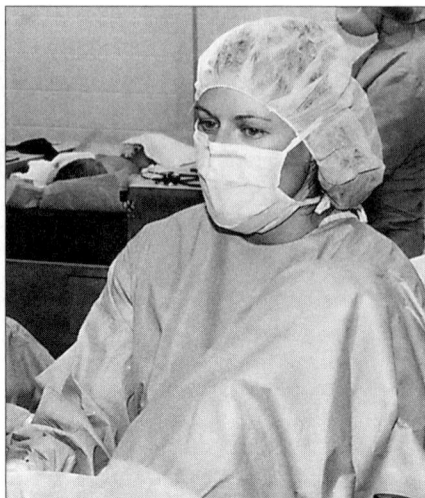

Above left, I am a medical student acting as a medic in St. Paul's June 1972 peace march during the Vietnam War. It was a rainy day, and all the medical students wore headbands labeled "Medic" and arm bands to identify ourselves during any medical moments. Above right, I have just delivered a baby and am attending to the mother. The newborn lies in the warmer to my right. During the years of my medical career, I will deliver over three thousand babies.

Below, after five years of undergraduate university and four years of medical school, I have graduated. This is my graduation day. It's huge! I opted not to wear a traditional cap and gown, as did more than half of my medical school class of 250. Thinking back on it, I can't imagine why it was important to do that, except that so many societal norms were in flux, and this was just more evidence of that. Eventually, graduating classes went back to cap and gown.

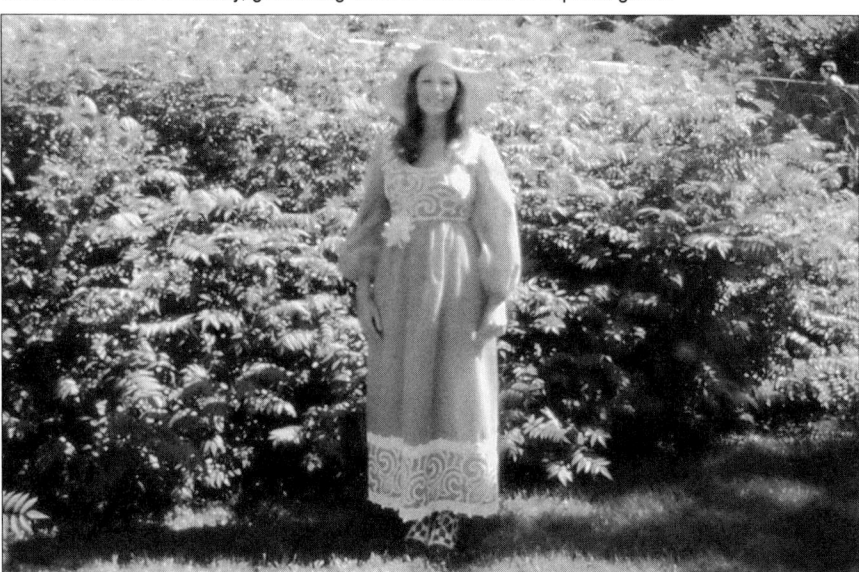

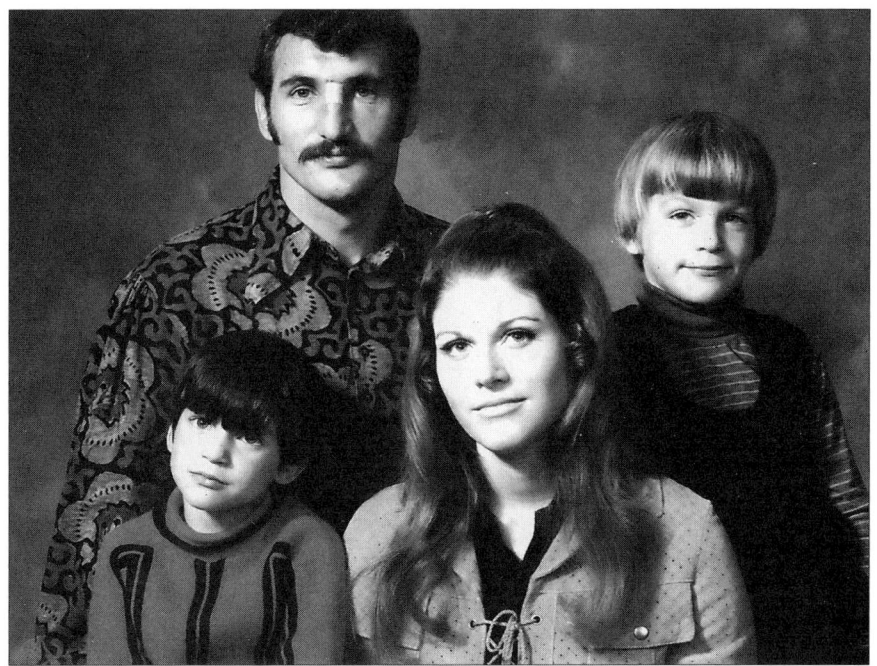

Above, this is our last family portrait before our divorce. Karl looks aged and beat up. The kids and I aren't smiling. Divorce was just six months away. Below, the kids are having a great time feeding the pigeons at a park in London. They sit on the ground, oblivious to the bird droppings. (I prefer not to sit.) It is a happy time.

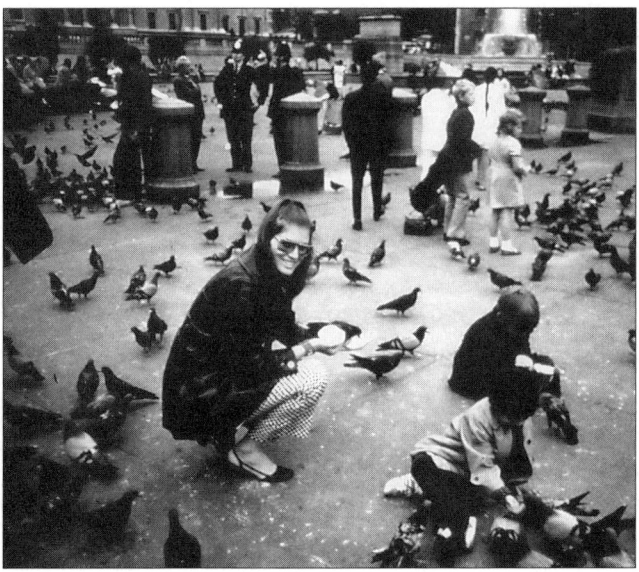

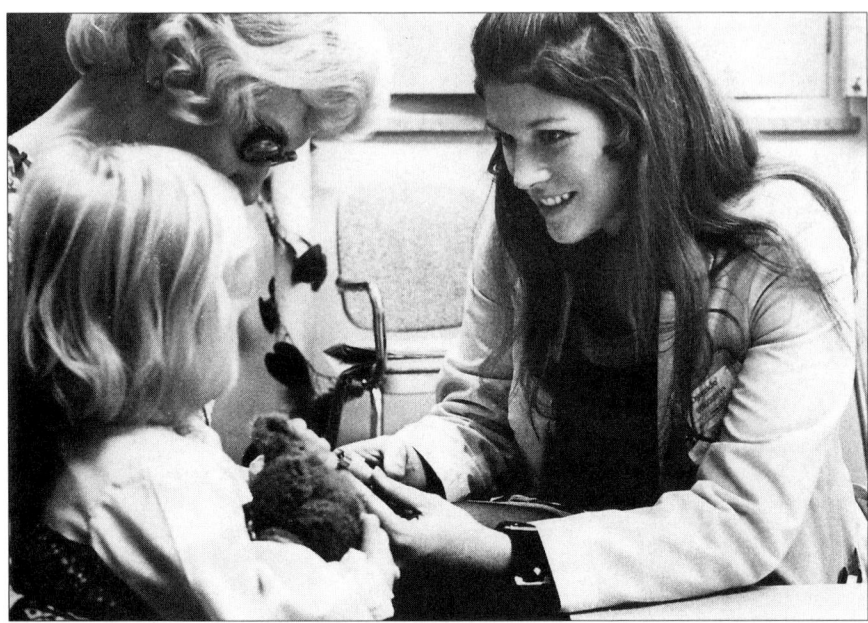

Above, I examine a young patient at the University of Minnesota Hospital. Below, teenager Kory enjoyed boating and fishing on the lake at our cabin. After our fun experience on vacation with Karl, the boys and I wanted to have our own place at the lake. We were able to realize that dream after I had been a practicing physician for some years. Both boys enjoyed water sports: boating, fishing, and especially water-skiing. They inherited their dad's athletic skills and excelled at football, wrestling, and track. From me, they inherited keen intellects and fine music skills.

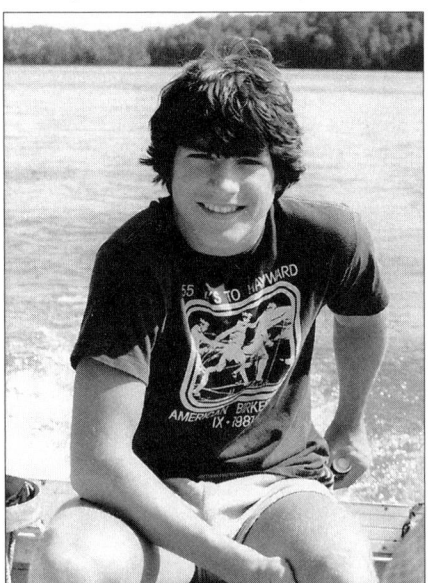

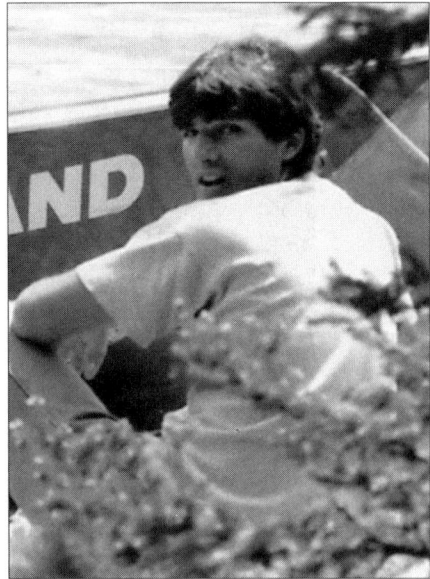

Chapter 16

The More Things Change…

*T*HE VIKINGS HAD A poor season in 1967 (3-8-3), but hopes are very high that they will do much better this year. The team continues to gel with their new coach and quarterback. An irony for Karl is that his old football coach from Drake, Bus Mertes, had signed on the previous year as the offensive coach for the Vikings. Karl is glad to have his old supporter back, though Bus is not directly Karl's coach this time.

The team dreams of winning the NFL title, which would mean they play in the Super Bowl, the game that determines the best team in all of pro football. But they must first win enough games to have the best record in their division (Central) of the NFL, then beat the winner of the other division for the NFL title. Maybe this will be the year. Eventually the Vikings will become known as the team that is always almost: almost to the Super Bowl, or if they do get there, almost winning the Super Bowl. The Vikings have never won the coveted Super Bowl trophy.

The families filter back into the Twin Cities from their homes elsewhere, we all get acquainted with the new rookies and trades, and everything settles back into the usual routine. Those players gone or traded are just so many ghosts. They are rarely mentioned or discussed. They've had their glory and ruined their bodies, and now they are just plain gone. This is the transient nature of pro football and, I suspect, of all pro sports. My thought is always that these men are just so much meat: useful until used up, then gone from the scene and scarcely remembered.

In time I will indeed see these guys give more than their all to this sport: they will give years of their lives. And before they die early, they will suffer severe degeneration beyond that of the regular population. This meat will pay a very high price for their glory. And those who go back to a regular life earlier will actually be the lucky ones. The longer one plays pro ball, the shorter his life will be.

And I have been struggling a bit about what I perceive as my own loss of identity. Since age twelve I have usually been compared in looks to someone else, usually some Hollywood star. When I was twelve, it was an actress named Dagmar. As Karl's wife, depending on my hairstyle or what I wear, I am compared to Raquel Welch, Katharine Ross (*Butch Cassidy and the Sundance Kid*), Ali McGraw (*Goodbye, Columbus*), and Amy Irving. Then, when I am overweight, everyone tells me I look like some good friend of theirs. Now, in 2010, I'm being told I look like Vanessa Redgrave. I finally just have a stock line to these comments because I know the people who make them mean well: "I guess I must have some kind of universal look. It seems everyone thinks I look like someone else."

This constant comparison of me to someone else in terms of looks doesn't particularly bother me. But what is bothering me as Karl's wife is that I seem to be increasingly identified as sort of an extra leg of Karl or a way to get to interview him or be even remotely connected to him. At work, remarks that should be academic or serious often end up with a discussion of what Karl or the Vikings are doing in the last game or the upcoming one. Just before I start medical school, a perfect example of this sort of thing happens.

The Burnsville Orchestra, of which I am not a member, knows I play and own a cello. They have a cello player who wants to participate in their next concert, but she has no cello. So they send a representative of the orchestra to my house to ask me if they can borrow mine for the concert.

This is a difficult decision for me. I have a very good cello, and its acquisition is a deeply personal story for me. When I was fifteen, I was about to become the first chair cello in the very good Boone High School orchestra. I'd been learning on and playing one of the school's cellos, which was adequate but a clunker. I wanted a better cello.

My teacher and orchestra conductor suggested I buy a cello from the Lewis Cello Company in Chicago. Of course, I didn't have the six hundred dollars it would cost, but I just assumed I would buy it somehow. So, I walked into the local bank at age fifteen and asked for a loan for the full amount. Everyone knew everyone in Boone, so the bank was aware I worked every day after school at a store down the block, and they knew my reputation as an outstanding student and a hard worker.

"Just how do you expect to pay for this loan, young lady?" asked Mr. Williamson.

"Well," I answered, "I'll give you twenty dollars a week, and often more, until it's paid off."

And just like that, they gave me the loan!

So with my six hundred dollars tucked safely away, I took the early morning train to Chicago by myself, then a taxi to the Rush Street building that housed the Lewis Cello Company, under the El. There the salesman opened wide the magical chambers for me, and I tested a Stradivarius cello, among many others. What a thrill and honor! Of course, I decided on a Lewis cello and case for exactly six hundred dollars and proudly left, lugging my prize under my arm.

I had some time before the evening train would take me home, so I went a few blocks away to the Parker House Hotel and had an exotic meal in their Polynesian room. It was all very heady. Here I was, fifteen, having just made an independent decision on my own cello, which I'd be paying for over the next year, now enjoying a meal at a unique, high-class restaurant. Then I got back to the train and headed home. This is the cello I've used ever since, through many orchestras and many solo performances, and it's very dear to me.

So it was with some hesitation that I loaned the cello for this one performance of the Burnsville Orchestra. I met the player and expressed to her the fragility of my prized cello. She promised to take good care of it, and she did.

The next week, the headlines on the front page of the Burnsville paper read: "Karl Kassulke Loans Cello to the Burnsville Orchestra." This is just one example of how I seem to be disappearing as an individual, and though I'm about to enter medical school—an extremely individual thing for a woman to do—I'll continue to feel as if I'm fading steadily into this invisible extension of Karl for the rest of our marriage. Even after our marriage ends, this issue trails behind me like a lost shadow. For a very long time, I will be known as the former wife of Karl Kassulke, and individuals will still want to converse with me about the Vikings years after Karl and I divorce.

✙✙✙

THIS PRESEASON is particularly special and unusual for me. Just before Karl gets home from training camp, I start medical school. I am one of fifteen privileged women in a freshman class of 250. It's difficult to explain the emotions I feel on the first day of school, knowing this is truly the beginning of the next very important chapter of my life. I know without a doubt that I have chosen a very satisfying career.

The required freshman classes are anatomy, physiology, biochemistry, and pharmacology. Of course, anatomy means what it says. We are assigned a cadaver, which we will spend the year dissecting bit by bit. In that way we learn every tiny structure of the human body, how it all fits together, and how it all works together.

In anatomy lab, the first day is a shock, partly because the unfamiliar and potent Formalin smell knocks us backward the first time we enter the room. It permeates so strongly that we all smell of Formalin until we can change our clothes and shower after every lab. Of course, the sight of a very dead, shriveled, and pickled old man who we must delicately cut to shreds is also disconcerting. Four students are assigned to each cadaver, alphabetically, and each quartet of four will probably forge the strongest bonds throughout all four years of medical school. Dissecting a cadaver is a very intimate activity, and those who share in it are a part of each other's personal medical school story.

Because we are all uncomfortable with this laboratory and the reality that this was a human with a story and people who loved him, we do what all medical students do. To relieve the tension, we make jokes and tell macabre stories. To an outsider, it may look as if we are disrespectful, but nothing could be further from the truth. It is the full impact, starting on day one, that humans, just like this one, will one day depend on us for life-and-death decisions. And all of us will be dead someday, just like this man. These realizations force us to confront our own feelings about death and human respect. The strength of this most unusual situation— one that most humans will not deal with until they are much older— causes the usual kidding around in an anatomy lab to relieve the tension.

At first, Karl wants to hear about this cadaver. It's such a weird concept for him to think about his wife cutting up a dead man. Plus he doesn't like the lingering Formalin smell on my clothes. I can tell he's a bit repulsed by the whole thing. After a few days he says, "Please, I don't want to hear this. Keep it to yourself, Janny." So I do.

As for the other classes, I've already had physiology and biochemistry with the medical students, and just as I suspected, the classes are identical to my previous experience, right down to the examinations. For this reason, my first year is very easy, as I'm basically repeating half of the classes. I'm absolutely certain I've made the right decision, though. I can't get enough knowledge of medicine, and I soak it up.

Kory is still just a year old, so occasionally, when it's not a lab day, I will backpack him to lectures with me, but that doesn't work out very well. He's not content to remain quietly attached to my back. He wants to run and play, so I give up on that experience after a few tries.

This is now the full-on hippie era, and much of this medical school class is very liberal politically. Some are full-on hippies who've attended alternative colleges and universities. Nearly everyone in class discards the idea of wearing a tie (if a guy) or a dress (if a woman). We are rainbow attired, casual, wearing sandals (open-toe shoes are forbidden, but we do it anyway), and many of the guys have long hair, though that's also forbidden in the medical school policies.

My particular group of four K's (from anatomy lab) and a few others become my closest friends. I don't really have to study much (except before tests), so during the freshman year I spend a good deal of time in the medical student lounge (or adytum), playing bridge or hearts with these guys.

By the time the football season starts, I'm going full steam as a freshman medical student. I quickly discover that with my photographic memory I can calculate how many hours it'll take to review all the materials that will be on a test, then drive to the university that many hours before a test and cram. This might mean, for instance, if I think it will take me eight hours to go over all the textbook and notes, and the test is scheduled for 9:00 a.m., I'll come to the study lounge at 1:00 a.m. and study straight through until the test. Then I'm set, as I can get a picture of the page with the answer on it for most of the questions on the test that I don't remember right off. Rose, my wonderful day-care provider, agrees to keep the kids overnight for me when I have to do this cramming.

⌇

DURING THIS preseason, one shocking event takes place. The call in the middle of the night proves to be a theme of my life, and I receive another one on our unlisted number. The phone rings at 3:00 a.m., and I answer it with a feeling of dread. The last call like this wasn't very good news.

This time, though, it's a man. With a peculiar flat voice, he says, "I watch you at the medical school and at the student union. I know where you take your boys to Rose's day care. I'll kidnap your children if you don't meet me tomorrow by the third column in the main room of Coffman Student Union at exactly 1:00 p.m. And believe me, I'll do it. Don't call the police, or there'll be worse trouble. I also know where your house is in Burnsville." And he hangs up.

My immediate reaction is again gastrointestinal. I race for the bathroom and have diarrhea. I have a stalker! And this is before such a concept is even a word. But clearly someone's been watching me and knows my pattern, and somehow he has my phone number.

I can't get back to sleep. My mind is very noisy as I sift through all the possibilities and dangers of this man. Something about the call, though, just doesn't ring true to me. With probably very foolish bravado, I make up my mind as to what to do. I don't even bother to tell Karl, who has once again slept right through the call. I guess this is a clear statement about the state of our marriage.

I don't go to Coffman Union the next day. In fact, I will avoid the building the rest of my medical school days. I've warned Rose not to open the door to strangers or to let the kids be outside. All is quiet, and I pick up the kids and drive them home at the end of the day quite uneventfully.

But just a scant moment after we've all come in from the car, the phone rings.

"Jan, I told you not to have the police there. Why did you do that? Now I'll really have to punish you." Of course, I didn't have the police there, so I forge ahead with my planned speech.

"You know what," I say with the sternest voice, trying to control any quaver as best I can, "if you think I'm afraid of some guy who masturbates while he calls women to scare them, you better think again!" and I hang up.

Fortunately, because in the future I'll learn just how dangerous a stalker can be, this particular stalker doesn't reveal himself to me again. Years later, in 1974, a most unsettling event occurs.

As a family physician in Shakopee, Minnesota, I'm required to rotate with the other doctors in doing the examination and care of mental patients admitted to the hospital by the court system for a seventy-two-hour hold. This three-day period is used to decide the disposition and forward-going care of these patients, whether it be a psychiatric hospital, a state mental institution, a prison psychiatric ward, or release for outpatient care. Most of the patients admitted to the hospital for this purpose don't have their own doctors, so we're assigned in rotation.

On this day I must see a man from Waconia who is a paranoid schizophrenic. He's stopped taking his medication, and his family has felt threatened by his behavior. So the nurse leads me down the hall to the locked room on the medical ward. Her shoes squeak as we walk to the very end of the hall. There she lifts out a ring of keys from her pocket and unlocks the doors to his room, first the outer door, then the inner. She introduces me to him, then turns with a loud squeak and exits the room, locking me in alone with him. I feel safe because the red panic button is right behind me. I can get help if I need it.

The man is wild-eyed, disheveled, and unshaven. He has a noticeable, unpleasant animal smell, and his long brown hair is stringy. I say, "I'm Dr. Jan Adams, and I've been assigned to make sure you have everything you need while you're here."

He looks me straight in the eyes and says, "I know who you are. I used to watch you at Coffman Union."

This is six years after that call in the middle of the night, but I immediately know I'm locked in a room with my stalker, and it isn't a good feeling. I have to contain my reaction to him somehow and disguise my fear. I can't lose control of the situation, if in fact I have any. Not only is this the man, he clearly has continued to stalk me, as I've changed names since that terrible call. Yet he still recognizes me. "I was hoping I'd see you. I knew you worked at this hospital."

Trying my best to be respectful but well aware that I might be in danger, I press the red button, and then I try to engage him in conversation. He's actually risen from the bed and is walking toward me, trancelike, around the bed.

"What's been happening in your life to land you here today?" I ask with a slight tremble to my voice.

I can hear the hurried squeaking coming down the hall and am holding my breath that the nurse will get me out of this room in time. The doors begin to rattle, and I know she's working the keys to get to me. When he hears this, he stops coming toward me and mildly goes back to sitting on the bed. The nurse bursts in, deep worry lines on her forehead. "Dr. Adams, are you all right?"

"I'm okay, but I think there's a conflict of interest here. I'm afraid you'll have to assign another doctor for this gentleman."

As I leave the room, he calls after me, "See you around."

I head straight for the doctors lounge, pop open a can of Tab, and sink into a couch. There aren't any other doctors around, so I just sob a few times, and then straighten up and get on with the rest of my day.

"See you around..." These are not comforting words. I never did see him again, but I kept track of him for a few years. All during that time, he was hospitalized at a state mental institution. At some point I just forgot about any threat from him, and that was that—I thought. When my son Kory read the first draft of this book, he told me a very disturbing story, one he'd completely forgotten.

When he was a freshman at the University of Minnesota in 1986, feeling a bit alone and homesick, he was crossing the bridge over the Minnesota River, getting off near Coffman Union. Suddenly a strange, disheveled man with dark hair and a nervous tic of twitching two fingers on his nose approached him and started peppering him with questions about me.

"I know you're Kory Kassulke, and I know all about your mother. She used to be Kassulke, and now she's Adams. She did a lot of research here. Now she lives in Shakopee. Tell me more about her. I need to know everything about her."

Kory couldn't shake the man off and was thoroughly frightened. "How could you possibly know my mother? Why do you want to know about her?"

"I have to know! You have to tell me!"

Kory, in a bad state of mind to begin with, began to cry and ran as fast as he could to get away from this man. He never saw him again and never told me about it until he read my manuscript and realized I may have had a stalker all those years.

So very early in my medical school career, more adventures begin. And shortly after school begins, the 1968 football season arrives.

+‑+ +‑+ +‑+ +‑+ +‑+ +‑+ +‑+ +‑+ +‑+ +‑+ +‑+ +‑+

Chapter 17

Life in the Good Ol' Boys Club

*B*Y NOW I AM so very aware of how my life completely revolves around the cycle of the Minnesota Vikings schedule. Though my personal life is more ordered by children, school, and work, our family basically rotates through the same cycle every year. Off-season, preseason, and regular season.

So off we go again. High hopes, maybe more realistic this time, abound for a divisional championship at least. The fearsome front defensive four, the Purple People Eaters, are now a solid wall of trouble for opposing offenses. And new members to the offense have strengthened the team as well. The Vikings win their first four games, a fantastic start to the 1968 season. Then they lose a few, and then win some more, finishing the season at eight wins and six losses. This is their first Central Division title, but they lose to Baltimore in the conference playoffs for the NFL championship, so they don't quite make it to the Super Bowl. Again.

But the usual postgame parties during the season are getting more and more out of control. And as a well-established and increasingly successful NFL team, the Vikings begin to attract out-of-town celebrities to many of these gatherings. At one such party, a pungent, smoky haze drifts through the conference room at a downtown hotel, and the special celebrities here tonight are the singing group the Fifth Dimension.

This group is currently rocking with "Aquarius," "Wedding Bell Blues," and "Up, Up and Away," to name a few of their hits. They and their music are known everywhere. All five of them are at this party. Tomorrow night is their concert, so they're up for some fun tonight.

I'm wearing red suede bell-bottom pants and a red silk shirt covered by a purple suede tunic (pseudohippie, with my regrown waist-length hair cascading down my back). I'm not much of a party person and usually end up finding someone to talk to in a quiet area. But this party is memorable for me because it turns out Marilyn McCoo, the lead female singer for the group, doesn't much like big parties either and seems to recognize the same trait in me.

So she wanders over and comments, "Wow! I really love your outfit!"

From there we find it fun to talk with each other and spend much of the evening in conversation. A lot of what we talk about is the nature of celebrity and what it does for a person and what trouble it causes. Both of us recognize how lucky we really feel at our unusual lives and also are aware of the problems that come with our celebrity status.

The team has finished in first place in the division but lost the playoff game that would have sent them to the championship. At this time there's something called the Playoff Bowl. It's held in Miami after the NFL championship game, and the contenders are the two teams that lost the conference championship games. The game is about third and fourth place, and the players get a financial bonus for playing this game: two thousand dollars for the winners and one thousand dollars for the losers, which is a healthy up-tick in our income.

I'm excited about spending a week in exotic Miami. There are jai alai games and dog races to attend, and we try to figure out how to bet. We go deep-sea fishing on a very large boat that carries several players and their wives. The water is rough, and I am nauseated the entire time and not interested in fishing. The best sights are all these big, strong men, players and coaches, hanging over the edge vomiting. I wish I had some film footage of that!

The ocean, beaches, sunbathing, and shopping fill the wives' days, as well as sightseeing all the way up to St. Augustine. There are fabulous parties every night with exotic food and glamorous people and places. The men sarcastically call this game the "toilet bowl," and their play is listless at best, though the game is nationally televised. The Vikings lose to the Dallas Cowboys, 17–13.

⁓

BACK IN Minnesota I continue to play bridge games with the Vikings wives in addition to medical school and research. During the medical school year, I will only work twenty hours a week in the lab.

At bridge club I'm now the medical expert, and much of our conversation centers around medical questions. Of course, I expound on what I know, but I urge them to see their doctor since I have little practical skill as yet.

The media coverage of our family continues, and to all outward appearances, we seem to be the Cinderella couple: the doctor and the jock. Kurt and Kory are now included in the articles and photos, and Kurt even models an adorable winter coat and leggings for a kids' fashion show at Dayton's Department Store. As payment, he is given the outfit he modeled, which is worth two hundred dollars! This is so over the top at this time. The outfit looks like something a wealthy English aristocrat's child might wear. It has a brown wool polo-looking cap with leather trim, a brown knee-length coat of wool and leather, and brown wool leggings with leather shoe covers. It's adorable, of course, but Kurt is growing so fast he only wears it a few times before it joins the endless pile of too-small clothes.

Of course, things within our marriage are not as they might seem to others. While I am not distant or cold to Karl in public or private and would never fight in public—even if Karl would actually fight—I am definitely more satisfied with school and my friends there than I am with my marriage. It doesn't really seem to matter all that much to Karl, as he is gone so very often. His drinking and drug use continue at an ever-increasing rate. And his football skills remain at a very high level for the team. He's somehow able to pull off living on the dangerous edge of life, hovering between health and death, while playing his heart out on the field. This is actually something many players do in the late sixties, but when I think of Karl in terms of this, I feel oddly certain he will not survive his habits.

Then the usual thing happens again: a phone call in the middle of the night. This time Karl isn't even home. It's two o'clock.

I pick up the phone to be screamed at yet again by a weeping woman. She says her name is Mary, and she's with Beth, who's crying hysterically in the background. "Your husband's been having an affair with Beth! Do you know that? And he promised to marry her!"

This time I don't have a visceral response. This is getting old, and I find myself wondering why Karl feels obligated to tell his conquests he will marry them. I'm pretty sure he could get them into bed anyway, but I will never know the answer to this question.

"And now he's broken up with her. He just left here, and I think you should know what he's done to her! He promised!"

I hang up the phone without comment, and it doesn't ring again. There are no more nails to put in this marriage coffin, but I confess to making a decision. If we have an open marriage, then so be it. Two can play that game.

Over the next several months, I will have flirtations and two short affairs. From this I learn many things, among which are, first, sex with other men is just as painful as it is with Karl. In fact, it's more painful since the act invariably lasts longer than the thirty seconds I'm accustomed to. Second, while flirtations might be fun, affairs are another thing. Clearly, my hopeful expectations of once again being cherished and having a special intimacy don't work well when the situation is an illicit affair. Instead, both affairs cause me great sorrow by forcing me to look at what everything in my marriage has come to and how very sad I am. It quickly becomes clear to me that affairs are not going to relieve me or shore me up or make me happy, so I end that particular activity until my senior year of medical school.

Fortunately for me, there is a unique study going on with the medical students that I become a part of. One of the deans of the medical school, Dr. Pearl Rosenberg, has an ongoing study with a "randomly selected" group of medical students. This group meets once a week for discussions with Pearl, who is a psychologist. The point of her study is to evaluate how medical school may or may not dehumanize medical students. It is part of a reevaluation of the way the medical school meat grinder seems to take perfectly nice people and turn out so many callous, arrogant, thoughtless physicians. This study is in response to patient complaints about many physician behaviors, and the results of the study will revolutionize medical school education.

We are not the first group Dr. Rosenberg has pulled together in this way. This study continues for many years. This group offers the chance for all twenty or so of us to vent about our difficulties with various aspects of medical school, our relationships, and other situations created by the demands of our education. I don't have a great deal of complaints about the medical school and generally don't feel comfortable speaking plainly about my problems with Karl in front of others. And although I am clearly a woman in a man's world, I'm usually not patronized or treated poorly or with disrespect—no more than a male medical student—as many of the women students complain that they are.

I assume it's because I'm a special case, a celebrity. But I also know it's because I'm not a strident women's libber, as many of the other women are. It feels more important for me to live the life of a liberated woman rather than to bitch about it, given the obvious advantages I seem to have.

But I enjoy the opportunity to be in this group and gain a great deal of insight into group dynamics and individual dynamics and thought processes. For me, the group helps me psychologically and teaches me many valuable skills. Huge benefits will come to me from this association that will last my entire life.

Perhaps the most important benefit for all of us in the group is that Dr. Rosenberg makes herself available for private counseling at any time to any of the students in her group. I'm hurting, though supremely successful in the eyes of most, and I'll use this opportunity to have my first experience of being counseled. Dr. Rosenberg becomes one of my most important mentors, as well as my friend, until her death in 1998. She quickly recognizes my unique challenges and my need for support, though they aren't apparent to anyone else. For the rest of my medical school years, she will counsel me, support me, advise me, force me to look at my life and my decisions, help me to understand my motivations, and always be there in a way no other person in my life is.

Besides all of the above, she models for me how to be an effective, useful, and compassionate counselor and healer, a skill family practitioners need to perfect in order to be complete doctors. And from the knowledge she gathers from her ongoing groups, the medical school begins to make sweeping changes to its curriculum, starting with the freshman year, to try to turn out more human and humane doctors. Pearl will nominate me as the medical student representative for the new curriculum development committees, so before the end of football season, I am already deeply involved in the core activities of the medical school staff.

This curriculum development committee is made up of all senior-level medical school faculty members, plus me as the student representative. The result of this is that I am privileged to work with and know many of the professors and deans of the medical school, often before I encounter them as my teachers. It's a heady time.

The first task for the new curriculum committee is to decide whether or not students need actual grades in medical school or if a pass-fail system would be better. The decision is to go with a pass-fail system, recognizing that all students in medical school are already outstanding academics who've been chosen at a ratio of one out of every two hundred applicants. This new system of grading is only partially implemented while I'm in medical school. Some professors just cannot give up the idea that competition for the highest grades is important.

The next task is to somehow introduce students to actual patient contact much earlier in their education. In the current system, students may not interact medically with a live patient until their junior year. Studies suggest this may be one of the reasons such arrogance and cynicism develop regarding patients by the time the school turns students loose on the populace.

So a new system is set up that goes into effect at the end of my first quarter of medical school. A cadre of practicing physicians in the community agrees to allow medical students to shadow them half a day a week. This proves very helpful in introducing students to the real world of patient contact much earlier in their education, and it does make a difference. This activity also helps us all to see, in a very concrete way, why we are beating ourselves up to get through all this extra schooling.

I am assigned to shadow an older general practitioner (the specialty of family practice has not yet been created) in Shakopee. It's the late sixties, and Dr. Bror Pearson is already elderly and has a daughter who is in my medical school class, so she and I become friends through this connection. Dr. Pearson is one of the original doctors in Shakopee, and at this time he has a very active practice. I find myself looking forward to the weekly trip to Shakopee to see patients with Dr. Pearson, and I also discover, for the first time, how very easy it is for me to establish a good rapport with these patients. I'm comfortable and interested in them, and they respond very well to me, though a woman doctor is something quite unique for most of them.

At the same time the medical school curriculum committee establishes this patient contact experience for freshmen medical students, it also arranges a six-week course for senior medical students that works the same way, except the student will shadow a local doctor every day, 24/7, for six weeks. This course, which I help to create, will prove to be life changing for me in my senior year.

Probably the most astounding curriculum change will require much planning and trial courses before it becomes part of the curriculum in two years. This is a course designed to address the fact, clearly shown in studies, that doctors have virtually no education regarding sexual behaviors and attitudes. As a result, they are very uncomfortable addressing this important aspect of their patients' lives. The results of ignoring or avoiding sexually weighted questions can be devastating for the patient. Misdiagnosis of sexually transmitted diseases, failure to note psychological problems or marital problems that are sexually related, missing pregnancy as a possible diagnosis, and difficulty accept-ing alternative sexual behaviors are all the result of absolutely no expe-rience or education on how to deal with these issues.

Quite by invitation only, I will now become an expert in human sexuality, so much so that I will in time be interviewed as part of an all-star panel for the *Journal of Human Sexuality.* The topic is foreplay. The recent landmark studies of William H. Masters and Virginia E. Johnson have opened these doors of interest by the medical school, and all of America is rethinking sexual attitudes and mores.

So a groundbreaking course in human sexuality begins to take shape, and this course is something quite new for the staid medical school community. Eventually, though, it will be adopted by most med-ical schools as an integral part of their curriculum. For now, creating it provides me with some interesting adventures over the next few years.

The first task is to decide on the process of helping students assess their attitudes toward sexual issues and to desensitize them so they can openly and easily discuss sexual matters with their patients. We are partly aided in our work by the Glide Foundation of San Francisco (of course), which provides us with personnel and materials for the course.

For the rest of the year, I'll attend several weekend sessions designed to help us pick out material for the course. We've decided that for an en-tire day the course will be a radical immersion into films depicting every form of the human sexual spectrum. Following that, the next day will consist of all-day group sessions to discuss and bring to the front issues the students may have regarding the previous day's material. The final goal is to create a freedom of speech regarding sexual issues so that the doctor-patient relationship may be open in this respect.

What all this means is that on Saturdays, for much of my freshman year, I'll bring my beanbag chair to the classroom and relax into it alone. We're encouraged to experience this as couples, and Karl does attend some sessions, but he's often out of town. So for the entire Saturday I will, along with deans of the medical school, heads of departments, and senior faculty, watch pornography of the most graphic nature.

Well, this is sure a new twist in my education. So far, I've never seen pornography of any kind, and now, before I'm done helping create this course, I will have viewed probably everything available, except snuff films. These films will range from sensitive lovemaking between real couples, to homosexuality of every kind, to amateur and commercial porn in every combination, including bestiality and masturbation.

Interestingly, viewing all these permutations of the human sexual spectrum actually does work as it's supposed to. Soon it's easy to discuss the most intimate aspects of the films with either gender, and we do all become desensitized by the activity. Of course, I would guess most get pretty horny while watching all this sex. I know I do get very pleasurable feelings in my pelvis, and Karl does benefit from it if he happens to be in town or at home when I get there.

For my freshman year, this is all we do for the course—we end up viewing hundreds of films and choosing the best and widest selection for the students to view in a single marathon, twelve-hour weekend day. Eventually, by my junior year, this course in human sexuality will be required of all students, which no one seems unhappy about. I will work much more on this course in my sophomore year.

The off-season has been unremarkable this year, with the exception that I'm gliding relatively easily through my freshman year of medical school. This isn't true for all, though. At least five students drop out, including a few of the women. It's hard for me to imagine making it all the way into medical school, and then finding that it's too hard or can't be accomplished. But it happens.

At the conclusion of this remarkable school year, I have good grades, am well known throughout the medical school and staff, and have been granted entrée into the inner workings of creating the curriculum I myself will be studying. And I absolutely adore the study and practice of medicine. Despite all of my challenges and problems, I feel like the luckiest woman on earth to have been accepted into this good ol' boys' club so completely.

Chapter 18

Med School Mom

*T*HIS SUMMER KURT IS three, and Kory will be two in September. I want them to begin nursery school in the summer. So I find a nanny to live in my home—we have a fourth bedroom in the basement—who will watch the kids and do the housework.

As for the cooking, my mom taught me to treasure very tasty meals and stressed the creative aspect of turning raw ingredients into taste-bud pleasure. Long ago, I began to collect cookbooks, and experimenting in the kitchen was a relaxing hobby. Now it's easy for me to create special meals and have them in the freezer, ready for any occasion or family meal. It's a delight to express myself creatively in this way while at the same time treating my family to the same kind of special food I grew up with. Whenever Karl is home, he raves about our meals. And Kurt and Kory will one day become superb and creative cooks themselves and will humble my own cooking efforts.

But for this summer the kids stay home while I continue to work at my research job. The nanny takes them daily to Betty's Nursery School in Bloomington. This is a kind of preschool with a structured academic-play environment, and the best part in Kurt and Kory's opinion is the swimming pool in the backyard.

Betty and her daughter teach the kids to swim, and swimming is a daily activity. Part of this is the astonishing diving practice the kids learn. Betty has a one-story shed right next to the pool, and she teaches the kids to climb up to the flat roof by a ladder and then jump (or dive) into the pool. This arrangement wouldn't pass any kind of code or day-care test these days. It probably was dangerous, but the boys adored it. They both remember this more than anything else about Betty's. They get a certificate of merit at the end of the summer for attending and for swimming. I have eight-millimeter films of their fearless jumping from this roof into the blue water below. They're having such little-boy fun. Freedom looks like the emotion radiating from their faces as they fly off the roof into the warm summer air, then splash down into the cool water.

I also enroll them in music classes at the MacPhail Institute of Music in downtown Minneapolis. The instructors work with young kids to introduce them to music and to strengthen their interest and musical abilities. The institute offers graduated classes, and the kids experience all of it as play, with rhythm instruments, keyboards, and all sorts of creative learning and fun. Classes are scheduled for every Saturday morning for the entire year, and I'll take the kids to class every Saturday for the next three years. While they're in class, I shop for family needs at the downtown stores, and then pick them up and hear their excited chatter all the way home. Both of them are musically gifted. This is already apparent at their young age, and they dive into every musical activity opportunity.

Karl isn't around much this summer. He's taken on a new activity: football camps for kids. He gets paid for this work and will be a coach at many such summer camps over the next few years. Parents and kids alike are thrilled to have pro football players at these camps. I imagine they pay a great deal for their kids to attend. The camps vary from one to two weeks at a time, and the Vikings players participate individually at camps in several states: Minnesota, Iowa, Illinois, Wisconsin, and South Dakota.

We also have a special vacation together this summer. One of my medical school acquaintances has a cabin near Alexandria, Minnesota. We decide to rent it for a week, and Karl, the kids, and I go off for a great family time together. This is my first taste of a traditional Minnesota lake home. Nearly everyone I know has a cabin at the lake (because there are over ten thousand lakes in Minnesota) and goes up to the lake as often as possible. This may be just a tent or camper on a patch of lakeside land, a summer cabin, or a fully insulated year-round home. It's all "up to the lake" or "up north."

This particular lake is ideal for fishing, and we catch plenty of fish for our meals, which I cook but don't eat. Because of the "muddy fish" I had been served in childhood, I'm sorry to say that the thought of seafood, lake fish, or shellfish will forever turn my stomach. I managed to get by with the muddy fish in Iowa by waiting for a moment when no one was watching me, and then taking the cap off the hollow tubular back of my chair. This was a perfect place to stuff fish or eggs, two foods that nauseated me. As long as I quickly put the cap back on, no one seemed to notice the stench around the back of my chair. But as an adult, I don't have to pretend to eat fish. I just don't.

The beach at this lake cabin is shallow, so the kids can splash around and make sand castles while we sit in the shade and play cribbage. Except for the leeches that seem to be particularly attracted to Kory, the entire trip is idyllic. The leeches keep coming every day, and they appear to consider little boy testicles a perfect spot to attach.

As a native of Wisconsin, Karl has a wealth of ideas for dealing with leeches. I've never seen them before, and I'm just flat out horrified by them, especially when they're attached to my little boy's testicles. So each day Karl rolls out a new remedy to detach them from Kory.

On the first day, Karl pours salt on them. This doesn't bother Kory, but the leeches quickly detach and disgorge his blood into a salty slurry. It's disgusting, and I ask Karl if there isn't some other way.

The next day, he applies a lit match to the leech. This is a bit dangerous, since Kory sees no reason to lie still during this. But it is very effective, though it also results in a bloody vomit from the detached leeches.

On the third day, Karl pours beer on the leeches. Once again they readily detach but expel blood into the bubbly beer.

The fourth day, he pours vinegar on them. The leeches quickly detach and retch bloody vomit. Kory is singing and chattering with the fun of it all.

Finally, on the fifth day I ask Karl if there isn't some way to remove the leeches without the disgusting discharge.

"Sure, but what's the fun of that?" he says. So he carefully slips his fingernail under the attachment point and slides it around the area until the leech cleanly comes away—without any bloody vomit. And that's how we remove the leeches for the rest of the vacation. In the future, I will learn that removing leeches requires caution, because squeezing them or causing them to vomit can transmit diseases such as hepatitis or HIV.

Something else new for me is that the giant orange shelf mushrooms on the trunks of pine trees are completely edible. I cook them in butter, and every day Karl and I gorge ourselves on orange mushrooms in a variety of forms: fried, in salads, in omelets, and pickled.

It's such a relaxing and idyllic week, such a happy family time that I can almost forget my painful pelvis and smarting psyche. At the end of the vacation, though, it's time for Karl to go to training camp, so I'm managing by myself again. A few days after he's gone, I'm at work when the nanny phones. It's a particularly disturbing situation, one I have to try to handle from a distance.

⁓

Both of our Siamese cats have been outdoor cats since our move to Burnsville. Plato, the male, has taken to sleeping on top of the open garage door during the day. This door is automatically opened and closed with a remote control. Karl's gone to training camp with one of the other guys, so his car is home and in the garage.

Little inquisitive Kory, not quite two but still plenty to keep up with, has managed to get in Karl's car and push the remote control for the garage door. The result is disastrous. Poor Plato had no time to react, and his head is crushed between the closing slats of the door.

"Jan Kassulke, please. It's an emergency!"

"This is Jan Kassulke. Can I help you?"

"Oh, Jan, this is Marie." She is crying and sobbing. "Something terrible has happened, and we don't know what to do."

I can only think of my kids and have a desperate, sinking feeling about what's coming next.

"Plato is dead and stuck on the garage door!"

This is the way she tells me, and I can't quite imagine what she's trying to say.

"What do you mean, he's dead and stuck on the garage door?"

She tells me the awful facts, adding that both Kurt and Kory are crying hysterically and the neighborhood has started to gather to gawk at the scene. It sounds grim, with blood and brains dripping down the door and Plato's body tightly trapped.

"What should I do? I can't get the cat out, and the garage door is jammed."

I think for a moment, and then suggest the only course of action available. "Call the fire department. They should be able to help you." I have huge faith in this fire department, remembering the gas main incident.

I'm terribly saddened by the loss of my beloved pet. Plato has been such a good and loving companion, and my enjoyment of the day is blunted. That evening my kids' trauma seems to be gone, though Kurt has quite a bit to say about the whole thing. He describes the same fire department I interacted with a few years before. The whole thing is very exciting to him, including the removal, bit by bit, of Plato's crushed head after his body was removed. Kurt's very clinical in his observations, and I wonder if he'll be an anatomy professor when he grows up. It's hard for me not to weep while he goes on with the weirdness of the day.

Mrs. Plato is still alive and will be a widow until her death at the age of eighteen. She and Plato had gone their separate ways a year before this terrible event. So at the time of Plato's death, he and Mrs. Plato have separated as a couple. They no longer groomed each other or slept together curled into a contented ball.

The problem arose when Mrs. Plato, in heat, apparently encountered another male cat outside. After birthing three litters of perfect

Siamese kittens with Plato, during which he behaved tenderly and so-licitously toward her and the kittens, she gave birth to her fourth litter: six perfect black kittens.

Plato seemed to know immediately these weren't his kittens. He re-moved himself from her company and from the care of the kittens, and the two cats were never together in any way after that. In the future I'll often reflect on this situation and how pets sometime mirror the lives of the humans around them. This is certainly a time when Karl and I are steadily growing apart, though our times together are still warm and in-timate. We will always love each other. I think that's clear. And we will try not to hurt the other. But sooner or later divorce will happen.

People will wonder why I didn't divorce Karl and be done with it since things were getting so difficult. Well, this is not a time when divorce is done lightly. Society highly discourages divorce and en-courages couples to keep their troubles to themselves. Second, I'm able to sublimate my problems and compartmentalize them because I'm so satisfied with my kids, my research career, and my medical ca-reer. Third, I strongly understand Karl's fragile instability, and I fear for his playing career if I divorce him. Fourth, there's still a part of me that really loves him. Fifth, I'm completely codependent by now, though I don't know this term or understand the implication that, of course, I would stay with him. And finally, we're such a public cou-ple that I don't want to deal with the negative press should we di-vorce. This proves to be an accurate guess. One thing that isn't holding me back is the need for Karl's money for my medical school studies. I'm paying my own way, so I'm biding my time—for what final event, I don't know.

⁓

KORY, THOUGH, isn't finished with his hijinks for the summer. A new home is going up next door to us, and the basement has windows that circle the entire house at ground level. One day Kory sashays over to this construction site with one of his friends from up the block. They each pick up a brick from the pile intended for the indoor fireplace, and they smash out every window of the basement, fifteen windows in all. Say what you will, they are thorough. There isn't a single piece of glass left in any frame.

This is an innocent time in America when kids can play freely outside without fear of molestation or kidnapping, so the nanny doesn't witness this glass caper until it's too late. She's not watching their every move, nor is the mother up the block watching her son. The nanny catches them just as they're meticulously and studiously finishing the last window. They're conferring between themselves about what to do next when she finds them, bricks still in their little hands.

"Jan Kassulke, please. It's an emergency!"

"This is Jan Kassulke. Can I help you?" I'm swallowing hard again.

"Oh, Jan, I don't know how to tell you, but Kory and his friend have just vandalized the house next door. Really vandalized it."

Well, we're talking about a child just a month shy of two, so I can't imagine what he could have done. But when Marie explains it, I am somehow not shocked. This little guy is just crazy about breaking glass.

Of course, I should've been shocked, as the builder is very unkind when he yells at me about it when I arrive home from work. He's already itemized the damage: nearly seven thousand dollars' worth of glass and frames. I'm now properly chastened. But I know, from my own experiences with house building, that he has builder's insurance, so I just apologize and comment on how unpredictable very young kids are and how glad I am to know that his insurance will cover the damage. He huffs off, but we're never held financially responsible for this carnage. Kory is too young, as well as relatively impervious to punishment, to really discipline much.

At the end of the summer, Betty's session is over for the year, so I place the kids back at Rose Embry's for the school year. I begin my sophomore year of medical school while Karl is still in camp. This year the subjects are much more clinical, and most will involve seeing patients to demonstrate one illness or anatomical situation or another. This might be on the hospital ward with our professor or in the classroom with all 250 med students gathered around. Subjects this year will cover things like pharmacology, neurology, gastroenterology, cardiology, surgery, pediatrics, and so on through the systems of the human body. We'll not have any direct responsibility for patient care as yet.

Within the first few weeks of school, four of us—two juniors and another sophomore and I—will hatch an idea to start a free clinic on the west bank of the university. At this time, the west bank is a true hippie haven, and drug-related and venereal diseases are rampant. Most the inhabitants are in their late teens or twenties, unemployed, living doubled and tripled and quadrupled up in cramped spaces, zoned out on drugs and music, practicing free love with enthusiasm, with a few of them attending classes at the university. These folks don't have medical insurance and don't receive any proper care for their serious health problems.

So we each identify specific areas of expertise we can use to get this clinic going. It will be called the Cedar Riverside Free Clinic, and we've secured a building on Riverside, a few blocks off Cedar Avenue. Half the building will be the clinic, and the other half will be a co-op that offers homemade whole-grain breads, nutritional supplements, and a variety of mostly homemade healthy foods.

Dr. Erskine Caperton, a rheumatologist on the university staff, has agreed to be our sponsor and will either mentor us himself as we see patients or have another staff person there. The clinic and co-op will be open seven evenings a week. The co-op has its own staff, and medical students, including sophomores, will staff the clinic. I agree to get together all the necessary equipment for the lab. This is easy to do as I'm still working in the laboratory area of the medical school. Other doctors donate medicines given to them as samples, so we have a full cupboard of treatments available. For the rest of my medical school career, I will volunteer at this clinic one or two nights a week. Usually, I will bring my kids with me after picking them up from Rose's. The co-op folks are happy to look after them while I see patients.

The clinic will provide me with more pathology than I will ever again see in such concentrated amounts. For instance, I'll care for the only cases of primary and secondary syphilis in my entire career. I'll see people with lungs permanently damaged by injecting the drug Darvon, something I don't even know about before this. Apparently the filler used with Darvon in capsule form lodges in the lungs and permanently scars them. I will see case after case of these issues, all in hippies—full-on hippies living the life. They are colorful, whacked-out, sick, under-fed, full of lice and crabs, and needing extensive attention. Dr. Caperton is a wonderful teacher, and I have a huge leg up on the rest of my classmates, because very few of them will ever have this kind of clinical experience.

This clinic continues long after I'm gone from the medical school. It eventually becomes a part of the medical school and is no longer free once the hippie years are over. The clinic morphs into a primary care clinic for teaching family practice, and it's still there today.

These are also the Vietnam years, and there's going to be a massive antiwar walk from the university to the state capitol. It's estimated there will be around ten thousand protesters. It's assumed this will be a peaceful protest, but medical problems can emerge, so the planners re-cruit medics from the medical school. I volunteer, as do many of my liberal friends in the sophomore and junior classes. We wear white doctor coats over our semihippie attire, with headbands, long hair, pierced ears, miniskirts, and rainbow-colored clothes. We have bright red armbands that say "Medic," and we know where the ambulances are parked in case we need them. We walk along with the crowd with an eye out for medical problems.

No problems arise that I know of, other than a fitful rain, so the whole day is an expression of massive good energy as the crowd surges along, both larking and serious about the issue at hand. I will take a photo of one of my friends sitting atop a street sign and another sitting atop an ambulance. My right hip hurts from the hike once we get to the capitol. It's the first time in my life I begin to notice a wee physical change due to aging.

+〜+

OUR GROUP meetings with Dr. Rosenberg have resumed on day one of our sophomore year. We are all well acquainted now. This is deliber-ately not a group of tight friends. We are liberals, conservatives, shy, outgoing, single, and married (me). We have little in common except for our shared experience in medical school. But I am learning experientially how to work with a group. This will be important for me very soon.

The curriculum committee also swings into high gear again to finish planning the course in human sexuality. This year we're going to have several tryout sessions. The attendees will all be medical school faculty and their partners (generally spouses). So this year we'll have one day of films to watch and the next day we'll be working in groups of ten or so to process what's occurred. We'll focus on any changes in attitude among the participants and on any new knowledge or revelations they might feel. We will want to know if they believe that this type of course will help them in their sexual frankness with their patients.

So I'll have nearly another year of watching these films, by now a prescribed set, not a new bunch each time. This will give me time—since the novelty has worn off—to reflect on the sexual revolution sweeping the country and how my own generation of women has missed this revolution. The films cause me to fully understand what I've not had in my own life and to wonder if I will ever have it in a relationship with a man.

Once again, Karl will attend a few of these sessions with me as my husband, and he causes a sensation each time he's there. In addition to his good looks, he's a celebrity, and many folks want to talk with him. Some of both sexes clearly hope to get involved sexually with either him or both of us. Neither of us takes anyone up on these approaches, but some are actually funny.

In one session, the head of a department in the medical school is lying on the floor behind me in his beanbag chair. My hair is very long at this point, and during the middle of the films in the darkened room, I feel my hair being moved a bit, then much more. I think someone has just shifted and don't initially pay it much attention. But the tugging gets more intense, as if someone is brushing my hair, and finally I turn to find this department head absentmindedly (perhaps) stroking my hair. He doesn't notice me looking at him at first, and then he drops my hair like a naughty boy caught with his hands in the cookie jar. This is a man who is my superior, who will be my teacher in just a few weeks. I tuck my hair under my body, and we get on with the session.

At another time, Karl and I are standing by an elevator at the end of the first day of films. A representative from San Francisco is there beside us. He suggests perhaps we'd like to have a threesome with him: Karl, me, and him. We politely decline and giggle together about it later.

There's often a party at a faculty home at the end of the first day. I don't usually attend unless Karl is with me. These parties can get wild, as there's a strong sexually charged atmosphere, and I'm not interested in sexual experimentation at this time. But there are at least two marriage breakups and affairs that are the result of these parties. These circumstances become the subject of much gossip among the staff, and the outcome of all this experimentation is not always positive. I'm glad I've steered clear of it.

The really interesting part for me this year will be the second day of the human sexuality courses. I find I must be a group leader, although I lack any real training in this other than my observations of Dr. Rosenberg and her techniques. I will play this role with such couples as the dean of the medical school and his wife and many other department heads and officials. It turns out that I am not nervous about this, and the discussions are productive and focused. Once again, I am incredibly lucky to have a depth to my education that few medical students experience.

By the end of the year, the course is set and will be a required course for the students beginning the next year. I never actually take the course, but I'm given credit since I've attended about twenty sessions. The course continues to this day and has spread to most of the medical schools in the country. I like to believe we made a difference in the lives of countless Americans whose sexually related problems had been habitually ignored by previous generations of doctors.

Such situations will arise with remarkable frequency in my future years as a family practitioner. I believe I was able to handle them without judgment or belittlement thanks to this course. I learned that there's an infinite variety of behavior along the spectrum of human sexual activity, and it was a valuable lesson. For instance, when a patient I'll call

James came in one day and said his wife needed to see me right away, I asked, "What's the problem? Why isn't your wife with you today?"

I was also caring for his wife and knew her to be suffering from massive obesity at four hundred pounds. She was not yet experiencing many complications because she was still in her twenties.

"Well, I wanted to talk with you first about her problem."

"Okay, James, what's up?" I assumed we were going to talk about her weight.

"Well, she sits on cats."

I just looked at him, struggling to keep my poker face. "I don't think I understand. What do you mean, she sits on cats?"

"Just that, and it kills them. The neighbors are starting to complain."

"Why are the neighbors complaining?"

"Well, she's killed all the cats in the neighborhood."

I think I was a bit dense, because I asked, "But why is she doing this?"

He looked at me like I was stupid, then said, "Don't you get it? The cats struggle a lot before they die."

Finally it occurs to me what he's trying to tell me: his wife is getting off on the struggle under her bottom as these cats die. Talk about working hard to be nonjudgmental! At this point I became absolutely certain I would never see it all, and I have been right about that.

This poor woman did eventually see a therapist. I have no idea if she stopped sitting on cats. As often happens, when individuals feel great shame for their actions, they stop coming to see a particular doctor.

―✦―

BEFORE I mention my first experience in assisting in surgery during my surgical rotation, I have to explain the practice of pimping. This is a common medical school activity in which a more senior person— either resident, staff, or intern—skewers a junior medical student with an obscure medical question that few can answer. Pimping is best performed when there is a group present so as to provide more pleasure for the senior person at the discomfort when the question can't be answered. This is such a common situation that it occurs daily to all of us.

But it's very difficult to pimp me. I usually know the answer, so I am generally left alone, as my reputation precedes me. It isn't any fun for the questioner if the one being pimped knows the answer. Pimping occurs in all arenas of the students' life. It goes on all the time, and everyone is anxious that a question will asked at any moment.

One of those arenas is the operating theater. During my sophomore year, I'll have my first experience in surgery. For me, this is almost a religious experience. As a medical technologist, I have sat in the glass dome above the operating theaters and watched Dr. C. Walton Lillihei do the first open-heart surgeries and Dr. John Najarian do the first kidney transplants. But I was outside the room. Now I'm to be admitted to the actual surgery.

This is a hallowed area of healing, where the full skills of doctors are put to precise use to bring about recovery. Everything is sacred there as far as I'm concerned. First the OR (operating room) nurse spends an hour with me, teaching the lengthy hand scrub and sterile donning of surgical scrubs. She instructs me in my behavior in the room. I'm to stand at the far end of the table, near the patient's feet. From there I will pull on a retractor (a flat, hooked steel blade that pulls the wound open for the surgeon to see what he's doing). I will not speak unless spoken to. There will be several other more senior students, residents, and interns present, plus the attending physician, the surgeon.

I go through the routine very carefully. I enter the room, which is, as I've imagined, quiet. There are only the scurrying sounds of the nurses and anesthesia personnel as they prepare everything, also the clinking of instruments as they're placed on the movable table to be available for the nurse who'll hand them to the surgeon. I'm gowned and gloved and take my place at the end of the table.

The operation today will be a gallbladder removal, and I've thoroughly studied my anatomy and pathology books regarding the gallbladder and pancreas so I can quickly answer any pimping. I'm absolutely certain I'll be pimped.

The surgeon enters, and the operation begins. I'm truly in awe. This is the center of a secret healing society, and I'm privileged to be here today. The surgery proceeds. I'm pulling hard on the retractor. I can't actually see what's happening, because there are too many people in front of me. I'm waiting for the pimp question. I imagine it will be, "Tell me, Ms. Kassulke, what is Courvoisier's sign?" I know the answer: it's the painless swelling of the pancreas in the area where the rib cage joins in the abdomen, seen in pancreatic cancer.

And the moment does indeed arrive. The surgeon looks up, directly at me. "So tell me, Ms. Kassulke..." I tense, hoping I'll know the answer. "Who do you think will win the Vikings game this weekend?"

This sums up the blessings and the curse of celebrity all wrapped together in one moment.

⌇

BEFORE THE sophomore year ends, there will be one final notable event. In pharmacology, the rules for attendance are clearly stated in a written handout. These class rules are absolute, and the professor states many times that his students must adhere to the rules inscribed on the paper. A student's grade each quarter will consist of two midterms and a final exam. It is possible to miss one of the midterms and have the final grade be determined by the grades on the other two tests, if the student has given at least two weeks' notice to the professor. There are absolutely no requirements stated as to why the test might be missed, just the requirement for two weeks' notice. As long as this notice is given, regardless of the circumstances, no grade will be issued for the missed exam, and it will have no impact on the final grade.

The NFL sponsors another trip during the spring quarter, this time to Venezuela. Both Karl and I want to go, so I give the pharmacology professor four weeks' notice that I will miss one of the midterm examinations as well as one week of school. He is red-in-the-face angry at me for this and tells me immediately that he will flunk me for that exam if I don't take it. Flunking an exam would have a huge impact on the final grade. Apparently no one has ever tried to miss a test before, and especially not for something so frivolous as a vacation. So I show him his own written handout and ask why he would flunk me when it clearly states I can miss the test.

He grabs the paper from my hands, crumples it, and throws it in the wastebasket. "Ms. Kassulke, I am telling you that if you do not take that exam, I will flunk you for that test, which will then require you to get an A on the other two tests to even pass this course! This is medical school, you know!" He is very, very emphatic. I am not sure if his rage is because I am a woman student or because I'm impertinent enough to feel I can still do fine in pharmacology without this one test. This is one of the rare moments when I wonder if it's a disadvantage to be a woman.

Even so, I will not back down, and Karl and I go off to an exotic week in Venezuela. It is a wondrous week. We're there during carnival, and the sights and sounds are beyond unique. One day we fly to Canaima, a small airport in central Venezuela—the kind where the flies sit on the blade of a fan lazily spinning under the straw palapa that serves as the airport terminal. From here we wander into an impossible sight of waterfall after waterfall, and the sand seems to have diamonds in it, it sparkles so (this is actually a diamond mining district). We cavort and play all day here, along the edges, underneath, and in the middle of waterfalls. One very big guy from another team has dressed as Tarzan, and we take several amusing pictures of him climbing trees, flexing his muscles, and yelling the characteristic Tarzan holler.

Then we board a small plane that does a flyby of the spectacular Angel Falls, the highest waterfall in the world, plunging 3,212 feet. It spills over the edge of a sheer cliff into the Amazon jungle below and into the Kerep River. The falls are so high, much of the water becomes vapor long before it hits the ground, thus it is full of rainbows. The plane circles the area several times, and the scene is so magical I can almost feel cooled by the fine mist at the bottom of the falls and hear the roar of the water as it nears the edge of a mountain cliff and careens over.

There is such a cornucopia of new wonder, I don't mind at all that I'll have to really hit the books in order to pass pharmacology. The only incident that mars this trip occurs when Carl Eller and I are walking beside the busy traffic of carnival time. It's early evening, and the throb of tropical bands comes from every direction. Suddenly, a car containing several passengers drives up to us and stops. In an instant the windows open, and they pelt us with rotten eggs, hitting us with several of them, so that we have to go back to the hotel and change clothes. I'm stunned. I'm just not used to being disliked. I learn through this incident that anti-American tensions are high at the time because of anger at Standard Oil for taking all the profits from the oil fields at Maracaibo in western Venezuela.

Karl enjoys himself enormously in Venezuela. The two of us still enjoy traveling together, and South America is very exotic. He wrinkles his nose when I return stinking with rotten eggs and honks cheerfully when I tell him what happened. We are together most of the time during this trip. It is clearly developing that our best times together are when we are away from the pressure cooker of celebrity. Karl acts more like the man I married, and I imagine I'm much less tense and more warm as a result.

All things must end, though, so after this amazing trip, it's straight back to school for me. I study hard in pharmacology for the rest of the quarter, harder than I will need to for any other course in medical school. I ace both tests and manage to pass and get on to my junior year. Were I not to pass, I would have to repeat the entire year of pharmacology—something I didn't relish since this professor scowls whenever he looks at me.

Soon I begin to mimic his look, and this gives me some relief from the tension I feel until I see my passing grade. I don't think the professor ever forgave me. Fortunately, I didn't have to interface with him much more at school, but guess who ends up in my group discussion session after one of the human sexuality courses. He doesn't participate much in the discussion.

Chapter 19

Chinese Fire Drill?!

*H*OPES AND TENSIONS ARE high for this ninth season of the Minnesota Vikings. After winning the Central Division championship in 1968, and with a very experienced team now, maybe this will be the year we make it to the Super Bowl. The energy of possibility is everywhere. Everyone can sense some difference, some hyperexcitement missing in previous years. I've watched all the Vikings games, either on television or at the Metropolitan Stadium, and I can feel this new enthusiasm. This just might be the year.

Everyone is chanting "forty men for sixty minutes" the full season. But the season opens with a narrow loss on September 21 to the New York Giants, 24–23. Everyone is a bit quieted by this, but their spirits still are high for a magical season. The team overcomes this first loss and goes on to win the next twelve games for a record at this time for consecutive games won by any NFL team.

Now we are all in a true frenzy. This is really it. Cheering has changed to screaming at the games. Beer is getting poured all over people when there's a good play. Fans are standing, jumping, climbing into human pyramids, and following the cheers of the cheerleaders. The crowd raises their fists in victory with every touchdown. Of course, so many things can still go wrong at any point, but we're all high on the potential of the season. And Karl's had many great plays, as usual, as have most of his teammates.

On December 21 the Vikings have their second loss of the season at Atlanta, but they win their second consecutive Central Division championship with a 12-2 record. On December 27 they must play the Los Angeles Rams for the Western Conference Championship at Metropolitan Stadium. It is the most exciting game I can ever remember attending. The outcome is so critical in order to get to the Super Bowl, and the Rams are a very fine team. But the crowd is in an absolute ecstasy of screaming, jumping, and adrenaline as the game proceeds to halftime with the Vikings trailing the Rams 17–7.

By the start of the fourth quarter, the lead has been cut to 20–14, and our hearts are pounding. We're so sure we can win this, and we must win. No one sits down for the entire fourth quarter. With some critical Vikings plays, which prevent any further Ram scoring, the game finally ends with the Vikings winning, 23–20. The stands erupt, and everyone is wild with joy, dancing and screaming. We've done it! We've done it! Our team has come through! We're now the Western Conference champions.

One week later, on January 4, 1970, the Vikings will play the final NFL Championship game against the Cleveland Browns before the merger of the National Football League and the American Football League, so it's a historic game. Next season there will be a complete realignment, with the two leagues forming the American Conference and the National Conference of the NFL.

It's also the last hurdle to get over before the honor of participating in Super Bowl IV. The Vikings dominate the Browns, winning 27–7. And that's that. The Vikings are going to the Super Bowl—finally! This is a huge accomplishment for a not entirely respected team that's just nine years old.

These postseason games are also important to Karl and me, as well as all the players and their families, because each playoff game means an additional check, whether the team wins or loses. The bonus money is much more for a win, but is still significant either way. For Karl, the bonuses by the end of the Super Bowl equal more than half his regular salary.

I drive by myself down to New Orleans to attend the Super Bowl. I'm very excited, and my failure to concentrate results in my being stopped by a patrolman in the South for speeding thirty-seven miles an hour in a twenty-five-mile-an-hour zone. I am issued a ticket and told I can't leave town until I pay the fine.

I have no idea what this means. I'm due at my hotel in New Orleans later that night. Karl is already there, practicing with the team. The game will be in two days—January 11, 1970—and I have to get there. It's already early evening, and this patrolman seems to be indicating I'll be in jail instead. I can't understand his language very well due to his accent. He ignores my pleas and tells me to follow him in my car. Surely the courthouse is closed by this hour.

We proceed down magnificent tree-lined streets—trees with moss hanging on them—to an old antebellum-style mansion. I'm alone and without my kids, and this feels spooky. I've dropped into an unknown part of the planet. The patrolman tells me to wait in the car. I still have no idea what's going on. Am I being kidnapped? Is this really happening? The patrolman rings the doorbell, and a black woman dressed as a maid opens the door. She nods to the cop, and then leaves him standing at the door. The cop gestures for me to come up on the porch.

Then a gentleman with a white, neatly trimmed beard comes to the door. He looks like the caricature we will in later years know as the colonel of the Kentucky Fried Chicken franchise. It turns out he is the magistrate and is expecting these evening visits in order to pay traffic fines. Everyone is very interested in my Vikings wife, Super Bowl story, and they're oh, so polite, but it's obvious they have no intention to let me go until I pay the fine.

The magistrate has a very official-looking desk in his living room, complete with a large paperweight that proclaims his name and office. My fine is $100. In cash, please. I have $110 with me, so I pay the fine. I have credit cards that will get me more gas if I need it, so I'm relieved to get out of this town. It feels like a movie set or something, it's so clichéd, and there is a dark, unfamiliar undertone I'd rather not tangle with. I want to get out of there before a figure with a chain saw looms from behind one of those giant tree trunks. And my car is going so slow, he could probably catch me on foot.

The rest of the trip on those pre-freeway roads is without incident, and I'm relieved to check into my hotel later that night. It's right in the middle of all the action in New Orleans, near Bourbon Street. My roommate, Marcia Kapp, wife of quarterback Joe Kapp, is already there. We won't be seeing the guys until after the game, so we have plans for the following day.

Beginning in the morning, we gorge ourselves on exotic New Orleans cuisine. We try to squeeze as much in as possible, from the beignets (small powder-sugar-dusted puff pastries) in Lafayette Square to the seafood gumbo (for Marcia), from the Mississippi River sights to the strange aboveground cemetery.

The cemetery, especially, is unique for us. It turns out New Orleans is actually below sea level, so if one digs in the ground, water wells up, thus preventing burial underground. I've never imagined such a thing. The caskets are all in little houses built above ground. Some are magnificent. Some are humble. All are completely weird to this northerner's eyes.

And we're also fortunate to spy a funeral procession marching in the traditional way with a brass band, singers, dancers, and mourners, all in colorful clothes and preceding and following a casket. The band is playing soulful blues. It looks like a wonderful going-away party to me.

That night, Marcia and I dress up and prepare to do Bourbon Street. It's the night before Super Bowl IV. The town is packed and alive with excitement, and we're going to check it all out. Very early in the evening we hear the old performers and music at Preservation Hall. This beat-up storefront, where we sit on cane chairs, is the epicenter of the blues and the fusion of black, Cajun, folk, jazz music that marks the particular American sound underlying much of the popular music of the world. We've heard the French, Southern, Native American,

African American influence in the Cajun music during the day, and tonight we listen to these simple, toothless, grinning old men as they play brass instruments and guitars in the quintessential blues style of New Orleans. They wear their souls on their sleeves.

Then we start checking out the crowded joints that populate the exotic architecture of Bourbon Street. Here the buildings have a strong French influence, with fancy iron railings lining balconies all along the way. Every restaurant and bar is packed, and the streets are filled with revelers as well. I've never seen anything like it, not even in Caracas, Venezuela, during carnival. Every time we squeeze into an establishment, we're noticed and introduced to the entertainers there. People want their pictures taken with us for souvenirs. We meet Pete Fountain after he finishes a fantastic set of clarinet jazz. He's humble and unbelievably talented. After a short chat, he goes backstage to rest up for his next set.

Soon we meet Ed McMahon, Johnny Carson's famous sidekick. Ed is attracted to us and even attempts to pick us up—that's obvious—and tries to keep his arm around one or both of us all the time. We tolerate this because the area's crowded, and it's very clear to Ed there will be no sexual behavior with us. When he discovers we're Vikings wives, he's doubly happy and hangs with us for a few hours, introducing us to celebrity after celebrity.

Probably the most notable is world-famous trumpeter Al Hirt. We meet him at his own club on Bourbon Street. I remember him best because his bottom lip is grotesquely swollen and because he is very heavy and a bit short of breath. I fear he won't live long at his present weight and obvious state of overcelebration (though he does survive until 1999 and dies of liver failure). He explains that he played in a parade recently and overdid it. It's the first time I will hear the word *ombudsure,* as he explains that if he uses his lips too much, they swell. Then he must recover the use of his ombudsure. He explains that this is the shape, tension, and placement of lips when playing a brass instrument like the trumpet or trombone, and that the lips have to be in shape, just like the muscles of an athlete. So he won't be playing tonight—no ombudsure. We leave Ed with Al, and they merrily pick up some women and go on their way.

Neither Marcia nor I drink any alcohol during this surreal evening, so we are clearheaded and able to avoid any problems. This is probably a good night for the husbands to be sequestered in a hotel, as there are thousands of predatory women roaming the streets, jiggling their barely covered breasts at every good-looking man. There is more public drunkenness, overt sexuality, and carousing than I've ever seen, even at the height of the Vikings victory celebration. I don't know what to make of it. I love this foreign part of America, but it's also a bit daunting.

Finally we walk to our hotel and go to bed. Tomorrow is a historic football game, and we can barely stand the wait. It's the last football game between the two different leagues—the NFL and the AFL—and the first Super Bowl for the Vikings. The Vikings are favored to win, and we believe they will. And so to sleep.

┼〜┼

We make our way the next day to Tulane Stadium for the big game (the Louisiana Superdome will begin construction the following year). Once the game starts, it's clear that something is wrong. The Vikings seem confused. Don't they understand the patterns of the Kansas City Chiefs? It looks like they don't. The Vikings fumble the ball, drop passes and kickoffs, and generally make mistakes—by players who usually don't make mistakes. And the big game-winning plays simply aren't there. I find myself wondering what the guys were doing last night. Did they drink or womanize too much? I'll never know, but they sure are off their game today.

Karl later quotes Hank Stram, the Chiefs coach, as yelling to his assistant, "Look at Kassulke out there! We've got him so confused he's running around like he's at a Chinese Fire Drill!" This quote hits the sports sections of all the papers and will follow Karl the rest of his career. He never does comment on the reason for his confusion, other than, "I guess they targeted my usual patterns, and played it different."

For whatever the reason, most of the team is off. By the end of the first half, we are behind 16–0. We never even get close to a touchdown or field goal. Marcia and I and the rest of the Vikings wives and fans are subdued during the halftime. The cliché—the wind has gone out of our sails—sure fits us all. We know it's hard to come from that far be-hind and win a game, especially one so emotionally charged as this one. But in the third quarter the Vikings' Dave Osborn scores a touch-down, and it feels like the momentum may change. The energy level comes up once again. Hope can be heard in our urging on of the team.

Then Karl's personal disaster happens. He misses a key tackle, and the player goes on to score. This apparently demoralizes the team, as they do no further scoring and lose the game 23–7.

We are all quiet and sort of mourning. We came into the game seventeen-point favorites and had such high hopes, but we did not perform well. For the wives, we know it will be challenging times for a few days. The guys will be in strange moods, to be sure.

The Vikings will develop a reputation as the almost... team after this. They make it to other Super Bowls in the future, but they don't win them either. They often almost win divisional championships or almost make touchdowns. The sportswriters don't know what to make of it. There's even talk of a curse on the Vikings.

I wish they'd won, but I'm so proud of this team anyway—and of Karl. But it feels a bit like Olympic champions who think they've failed if they get a silver medal. Second best in the whole world just doesn't count.

So the postgame party at the hotel is very subdued and discourage-ment reigns. There is none of the usual boisterous postgame revelry. Oh, there's plenty of New Orleans delicacies and alcohol in this conference room, but there's no feeling of celebration at all. It's sparsely decorated, with plain chairs for sitting but no tables. There's even a chill because the air-conditioning is too high. There are very few fans, perhaps be-cause the entire Vikings coaching staff and owners are here as well as the team, but it quickly becomes clear the guys are extremely disappointed.

Karl feels the loss was entirely his fault. Of course, this isn't true, and it's clear there are many on the team who also feel they're person-ally responsible for the loss. But he is despondent and doesn't want to talk at all.

Without a doubt, this is the quietest and most depressing postgame party I will ever see. At one point, defensive tackle Paul Dickson comes up to me and without any preliminary chitchat says, "When you've seen the top of the mountain, what else is there?" And he turns and walks off, while I puzzle what on earth he's talking about.

The next morning, I get back in my car and drive home. It takes two days because I'm driving very lawfully. When I get to our house, Karl isn't there. The boys are with their nanny, and Karl is off drinking, probably licking his wounds. He doesn't mention the game again to me, as we've probably discussed it all he can tolerate right after the loss. He has to be filled with alcohol to manage his pain.

This 1969 season is later chronicled in the film *America's Game: The Missing Rings,* an annual documentary produced by NFL Films, narrated by Tom Selleck, and broadcast by CBS on September 25, 2008. This Vikings team is listed as one of the five greatest NFL teams to never win the Super Bowl.

Karl and the team will mourn this loss more than any other game during the time I'm married to Karl. The media storm over the loss, the "Chinese Fire Drill" comment, and the many other missteps will haunt them all for weeks. It's like a funeral that never ends.

But, as usual, life goes on.

Chapter 20

Unexpected Opportunities

*T*HIS SUMMER I WILL need to go to school as well as work, because the medical school requires one extra quarter to complete the course of study. So I hire a baby-sitter at home to allow the kids to attend Betty's Nursery School again. As before, the baby-sitter also cleans the house and drives the kids to school in Bloomington. This baby-sitter will stay on after the summer, when Kurt will enter kindergarten at Gideon Pond Elementary School. The days at Rose's are over.

Both Kurt and Kory have been plagued with recurrent ear infections and strep throats. We've made many, many early morning visits to see Dr. Schaffhausen. Kory's eardrums don't rupture like Kurt's when he has an ear infection. Instead, Kory is suddenly miserable and cups his ears. Now that he is almost three years old, his vocabulary skills have developed so he can tell me when his ears hurt.

Dr. Schaffhausen recommends we see a prominent ENT doctor to discuss whether Kurt and Kory should have tubes placed in their ears and then have their tonsils and adenoids removed. They have been sick often and have had repeated courses of antibiotics, so I take her advice and make the appointment. When the day arrives, the doctor ushers us into his office. He listens for about sixty seconds to my story, then impatiently tells me he needs to examine the kids. He's heard the same story so many times before.

With that, he pulls Kory close to him, looks in his mouth with a tongue blade, then rubs his thumb and forefinger together near each of his ears, saying "Can you hear this?" with each ear. I am skeptical of this examination routine, as the whole thing takes less than a minute with each boy. Kurt answers yes to both questions anyway.

Then the doctor turns to me and says, "Yep, they both need PE tubes and their tonsils and adenoids removed."

I instantly rebel. This isn't a thorough exam or even a considered decision, and I don't want my kids to suffer needlessly. I have heard in my classes that some kids will outgrow this, and I make an immediate decision that I will not allow this surgery.

When I tell the important ENT doctor this, he gets very snippy with me. "So I guess because you're in medical school, you know everything now."

I answer, "I'm sure I don't know everything, but I know what's best for my kids, and they aren't going to have this surgery now. If they need it later, I'll chose a different doctor—one who takes the time to examine them properly and to talk to me about options."

He storms out of the room, and we leave. Both boys do eventually grow out of the problem and have fine hearing. Both will become superb musicians and singers. I will often wonder if I would have changed their voices by removing part of their resonating chamber. Kurt will become a re-recording sound engineer in Hollywood, and he will need perfect hearing for his job. For this reason, he will have frequent hearing tests, and there was no impairment by not doing this surgery.

As the years go by, the removal of both tonsils and adenoids will go out of fashion. The tubes and adenoids are still done, but it is clearly recognized that organs are in the body for a reason. Tonsils are finally studied and found to be an important piece in the immune system.

This is my first experience with a doctor who epitomizes why the medical school is changing its curriculum. He is arrogant, self-assured, and uninterested in the welfare of his clients beyond the bread-and-butter surgery he can perform to further his income. I am really upset at the experience, but it is a valuable lesson for me. I figure at least I know something about medicine. What happens to the folks who don't have this knowledge and must rely on such a jerk for their health care?

As the summer progresses, we have a minor uproar in the neighborhood. Karl has purchased a full-size trampoline for Kurt and Kory. This is before there are any safeguards, such as protective netting or pads, and the trampoline stands four feet off the ground.

I am aware of our vulnerability to lawsuits, because our family has a football player whom the public perceives as receiving a huge salary and because I will soon be a doctor. I am also aware of the inherent danger of trampolines—minor to major injuries happen all the time. Most importantly, I am also aware of several women in the neighborhood who strongly disapprove of me for working outside the home and for going to medical school.

Because of all these factors, Karl and I ask an attorney to draw up a document that releases us from responsibility should any child be injured on our property. We ask the parents to sign this document before their child uses the trampoline, and all of them sign except one family. This family is very insulted and responds by returning to our house with a document we must sign if Kurt and Kory use their swing set. Once again, I vow to live in the country when I have a choice.

Meanwhile, almost all the kids in the neighborhood enjoy the trampoline for hours on end. Kurt and Kory become very proficient at tricks and flips, and I become pretty good at it too. For all the years we have this trampoline, there is but one injury—a broken arm—and that occurs to the son of a doctor long after we have moved from Burnsville.

Karl is busy this summer with a few football camps. He is home just a few weeks before training camp opens, and then he's off again. Life is normal with us. He continues his headlong dash into disaster. I believe our marriage is damaged beyond repair, but once he gets back from training camp, I ask him if he will see Pearl with me for a few sessions of counseling together. I want to try one last time to help him understand my deep concerns.

He agrees. I know he loves me, but he isn't able to change. My concerns are the same as they have been since the first few years of our marriage, but they are magnified many times now. I am worried and unhappy about Karl's alcohol and chemical use, coupled with his self-destructive behavior, his desire to own a bar, and his wish to own a motorcycle.

These are the main topics of our marriage counseling meetings with Dr. Rosenberg. Karl is charming and funny and lighthearted. He isn't about to talk about anything serious, and Pearl isn't able to settle him down into a serious discussion, even when she talks about the possibility that our marriage may not last. Karl doesn't want to discuss this or anything else that feels threatening to him, and he doesn't. It is the first time the thought about the possibility of divorce has actually been voiced aloud, but he doesn't seem to have heard it. He is easily able to deflect all of my concerns with a laugh and a smile. He loves me, he says, and that should take care of it.

After two sessions, Dr. Rosenberg and I agree that the time has not been productive, and we abandon trying. This will be the first and last time Karl and I make an effort to save our marriage by unwinding the core of our difficulties. He goes right on with life as if the word *divorce* hasn't been spoken, and it is never spoken again until the very last.

⁓

My junior year of medical school is fascinating, and the courses now always involve patient contact. Many are directly on the wards of various hospitals. I am taught by interns, residents, and attending senior physicians. We are now learning real medicine and techniques, so we work directly with patient care daily. It is done by large topics, such as pediatrics, internal medicine, emergency room, and obstetrics-gynecology, and by subsystems, such as urology, neurology, gastroenterology, oncology, cardiology, ear-nose-throat, and so on. Each area is equally fascinating to me, and I see very quickly that I will want to do everything. That leaves me with one choice: family practice.

In my training, I'm collecting stories that every doctor and medical student will encounter in a million variations. For instance, one day on a surgery rotation, I learn how to thread a tube up a vein in the arm and directly into the large veins that pour into the heart. This is done in order to deliver large amounts of blood and fluids over several days. At this time, when there are overused veins or nonexistent veins, we learn to do something called a cut-down. This means using a scalpel to cut the skin and open a direct view of the vein. The resident teaching me will eventually become a prominent proctologist, but for now he's undifferentiated in his final choice. I do the cut-down under his instruction on a woman who is in a coma. As far as we know, she is unaware of anything happening to her. I successfully get the large-bore tube (catheter) in her arm vein and thread it up to her armpit, then I am called away and must leave the job to be finished by the resident.

When we return to examine the lady on our hospital rounds the next day, we discover that four pints of blood have been administered, and all four pints went directly into her left breast. So she has a left breast that is blue and gigantic. The resident pushed too hard on the catheter, and it jumped out of the vein and went into the tissue of the breast. When the resident took an x-ray to check the catheter's position, it seemed to be in the right place. This isn't funny, but it is if you remember the dark humor we all develop to cope with difficult circumstances. Fortunately, the blood will still get to the woman, just very slowly as it's absorbed through the tissue.

Also, we must learn to suture wounds, both from accidents and from surgery. There are many different points we must know and much to learn. To help us get used to suturing, we are sent to the morgue every day. There we must repair wounds on dead accident victims or possibly carefully sew up autopsy incisions using whatever technique we're supposed to learn for the day.

When I am on the neurology rotation, one of my patients is in an open ward at the old General Hospital. Minneapolis General Hospital is the finest teaching hospital in the Twin Cities, but it is a very old building—perhaps fifty years old—and the wards have open windows without screens on them. My patient is in a coma from a failed suicide attempt by strangulation. He has a feeding tube that goes directly through his abdominal wall into his stomach, and I am ordered to change the feeding tube one day, because it seems to be clogged.

When I bend over, I hear a strange clicking sound near the site of the tube. I don't know what this is. I'm totally puzzled. But my puzzlement is answered when I pull out the tube. It's covered with maggots, and they make quite a lot of noise. I'm horrified. But then the resident comes, and he seems pretty cool about it. Apparently this man has a chronic problem with maggots, and the resident knew it and was waiting for me to find out. Then he laughed at me.

From this I learn that maggots in a wound are harmless in general and may even be helpful. The maggots eat only dead flesh, so they actually clean up infected wounds. For this man, there is no way to get all the maggots out unless he's completely opened up, and that isn't going to happen.

A truly funny event occurs in the obstetrics clinic. One of our student group is very conservative, and he wears a tie every day at a time when almost no one dresses up in that way. We are being taught how to do a pelvic exam on very pregnant women by doing it from the side, instead of sitting at her elevated feet behind a privacy sheet. The point is that this way of examination is much more comfortable for the woman.

So it is the turn of this student to do the exam on a very pregnant woman who also has poor hygiene. He is trying to avoid the stench by standing as far back as possible, while at the same time inserting two fingers into her vagina to examine her ripeness and preparedness for labor and delivery. What happens next is a calamity for him, confusing for the patient, and hilarious for the rest of us.

Instead of pushing only his fingers into her, he shoves his tie in and pretends he is accurately feeling what he's supposed to. We all see what's happening and quietly snigger behind his back. When he tries to straighten up, he can't, because his tie is stuck. Upon discovering this situation, he faints on top of the woman.

My main problem with the way we dress is figuring out how to bend over patients for examinations while wearing a miniskirt and having very long hair. The men, of course, like to stand behind me while I struggle with this ridiculous miniskirt, and I decide I must always wear completely opaque tights when I wear it. Fortunately, this is a relatively brief phase, perhaps two years.

As for my hair, I quickly figure out how to tie just part of it back so it doesn't go in the patient's face or up a vagina. Such strange issues to deal with! These are uncharted waters for me.

⁓

THE ENTIRE year is fascinating for me. I truly love medicine and being in the role of a healer. It is so strongly the right choice for me. Everything comes to me naturally, and I enjoy everything I'm learning. I enjoy being with all kinds of people who have all kinds of problems. I like the detective part of carefully listening to the patient, assessing them in terms of body language as well, doing a physical exam, figuring out what's wrong, then putting together a healing recipe that will work. I learn to always find a way to leave a patient with hope and something to be done, even if it's a tiny treatment such as an aspirin.

It's a good thing I enjoy the year so much because I am at the same time somewhat depressed. This is partly due to my marriage situation and the hopelessness I feel about it. But it also comes from another situation.

In the last few years there has been more and more criticism about the use of amphetamines, and the drug is gradually being eliminated from any doctor's list of regularly prescribed drugs. Amphetamines are addictive, it's finally admitted, and thousands upon thousands of individuals around the world are struggling with the overuse of amphetamines and their negative consequences.

I've been listening to this new information in my classes. Although I have taken only one pill a day, I have been doing so for seven years, and I decide I will stop using it, which I do. This is a decision I make because of what I have learned, not because of any trouble getting my prescription filled. Dr. Stromme still gladly gives me a yearlong prescription each time I see him for my annual exam. I have filled the prescription at my local drugstore for five years without a problem. I just decide it may not be good for me and stop taking it.

This sends me into a depression. I am well aware of the cause and know this withdrawal depression will be over in a few months, which it is. But it is real, and I would have trouble functioning if I didn't have such a fascinating day every day.

I've also been learning the many other side effects of the drug. One is that those who abuse it (take more than one pill a day) believe they are functioning better. Actual scientific testing has proven that muscle function and coordination, in particular, are much worse when under the influence of amphetamines.

So one night, I am talking with one of the premiere halfbacks for the Minnesota Vikings. He's been dropping passes this season, which is something new for him. He had previously been a very reliable high scorer.

I gently begin to talk to him about his fumbles one night at a party. It's not like it's a secret. The news media have been complaining about it.

"You know," I say, "medical studies this year have shown that amphetamines cause the user to feel they are more effective in sports, but they are actually less coordinated. I'm not sure you should be taking all these amphetamines before the game. They might be affecting your performance in a negative way."

"You know," he says, "I thought the same thing. That's why I've switched to cocaine."

Again, this is a time when celebrities and sports figures do not have drug testing. The team may actually directly or covertly endorse the use of amphetamines, and the law is not likely to punish a celebrity for any alcohol or drug-related infringement or problem. Similarly, the media is not likely to report such problems either. So this player is convinced his performance is better now thanks to his switching from amphetamines to cocaine.

As for Karl, he is having a good season. It looks like another Super Bowl season, with a 12-2 record to win the Central Division title. But the Vikings lose in the divisional playoffs to San Francisco, so no Super Bowl. Karl is honored at the end of the season by being voted all pro by the sportscasters. That Karl would be chosen as one of the premier defensive backs in the entire country after his eighth season is fantastic. We're both so very proud of his efforts. He's a remarkable football player.

The honor means we will go together to Los Angeles for Karl to play in the postseason Pro Bowl game. This means another exotic trip for me. When we arrive, the cream of all the football players in both leagues is staying at the same hotel. Some are friends from previous travels together, others are new acquaintances. And some are surprises.

We party together, of course. I have always thought of one of our key players as a real straight arrow. No drugs, no drink, and no women. But I see him quite differently here. He is without his wife, and he participates in all three of these vices. I'm stunned and once again realize how very little I really know about the lives of these men I think I know so well. So many are probably living entirely separate lives in this arena, without the knowledge of their wives or families.

The parties are fascinating, of course. I have stopped smoking joints because I am nearing graduation from medical school, so I just observe. There is always a thick haze of smoke, perhaps even more than in Minneapolis. Hollywood celebrities are there and even some of the local football players, like O. J. Simpson, a college star. Everyone is dressed colorfully and expensively. People watching has become a favorite pastime for me, and this is rich.

But I receive a hard lesson when I go shopping on Rodeo Drive and realize Hollywood clothes are not made for tall, slender, size-ten women. They are created for size two and smaller. There is not a single item in any of the stores that I can wear. I can't figure out if the whole town is full of little people or what. Once again, I realize just how far off I am from the ideal woman, who apparently is short, tiny, and blond.

The game itself is played at the Los Angeles Coliseum in front of fifty thousand fans. It is not especially exciting, though the National Football Conference wins 27–6. I think I am less interested because all the very best players are here, and Karl's playing time is more limited than usual.

Back at school, as my junior year nears an end, I have another risky experience. I'm heading home. It's midnight, and my twelve-hour emergency room shift has just finished.

My car stops running at about Twenty-Fifth Street on I-35W. Cell phones don't exist, and there is no exit nearby to walk to. No patrol cars come by, and I'm trying to figure out what to do when a pickup truck stops and a grungy guy gets out.

The man offers to help. It looks like I need gas. It turns out I have a broken gas gauge, previously undetected. He offers to take me to a gas station and bring me back with the gas. I hesitate but decide to take a chance, something that would be most unwise by 2010. But these are more innocent times.

So I get in his truck and immediately tell him who I am, playing the football player's wife card. He responds as I hope. He unrolls the sleeve of his T-shirt, removes a cigarette from the pack stuck there, lights it up, then turns to me and says he doesn't believe me. Why would a Vikings wife be out here alone at this time? I finally convince him, and he relaxes, as do I. I have the distinct sense he may have planned something unpleasant for me until he finds out who I am. As it is, he does just what he promised. We get gas, go back, and pour it in my vehicle's tank. I give him an autographed picture of Karl (neither Karl nor I are ever without these in our cars), and he goes on his way. And I breathe easier. Saved once again by celebrity. Such a double-edged sword.

In the wind-down to my junior year, the associate dean of the medical school calls me into his office one day. Dean Albert Sullivan is the students' advocate, and he works tirelessly to make the medical school experience memorable and fulfilling for each student. He has an idea for me.

"Jan, you are ahead of the other students. We have an exchange program with the medical school in Cardiff, Wales, and I'm wondering if you'd like to do an eight-week elective there for part of your senior year."

The senior year in medical school is all electives. Students may choose all their courses for the entire year to fit with whatever track of medicine they plan to pursue. There are many courses to choose from, but I am indeed intrigued by this idea.

"We can find you a German au pair to help with the care of the kids, if you want to go. And we have a doctor there who will find you a place to stay while you study."

Well, Karl is gone most of the summer, first at football camps, then at training camp, so it seems a wonderful opportunity. I say yes!

Chapter 21

Summer in Cardiff

I SCHEDULE THIS EXCITING medical school elective to fit carefully with Karl's schedule, so he can tour England and Wales a bit with me before he has to return to training camp. I'll actually only be seeing him two weeks less than I usually do in the summer, given his schedule, so I feel it'll be fine. He has the usual football camps, the last one of which is in Iowa. Then he'll visit us in England.

I'm fortunate to be a university student. For students, the university travel agency provides cut-rate round-trip tickets to London's Heathrow Airport and returning from Paris for $125 each. I'm so thrilled to have the opportunity to explore the world some more as well as learn some different approaches to medicine.

One of the few people I've kept in touch with from high school, Melinda, is a nurse now married to a doctor. She and her family are living in Oxford while her husband completes a fellowship. So I make arrangements to stay with them for the last week of Karl's football camps. I'll explore the area around Oxford until Karl can come.

To keep everything running at home during my absence, we have a young woman staying at our house. She'll care for the cat and plants while we're gone, and Karl and I make plans to connect via phone the day before he comes to London to confirm everything. He is supposed to be home from the Iowa camp on that day, and he will call at a specific time. As soon as everything is confirmed, I'll pack up the boys the next morning, and we'll meet Karl in London. I very carefully give this written information to Karl, and I also jot it down for myself and tuck it in with my passport and papers.

The plan is for us to spend three days sightseeing in England as a family when Karl arrives, and then we'll take the train to Wales. Once there, we'll rent a car that I'll keep and drive the whole time I'm there. Karl will still have ten days with us to sightsee in Wales before I go to school and he heads back to training camp.

Packing for myself and two young boys for an extended stay is extremely challenging. I end up with three seventy-pound suitcases. Since Karl is gone, I must lug them into the airport myself and get checked while keeping track of Kory's wanderings. I end up tying Kory to the first suitcase so that he and Kurt are watched by the woman at the check-in counter while I fetch the other two behemoths. This is before wheels on bags make everything easier and before security police will drag off a person for leaving luggage unattended for more than thirty seconds.

Once on the plane, Kory kicks the back of the seat in front of him. I can't get him to stop. He's always wiggly like this. I try to reassure the man in front, who is rightly irritated, that Kory will soon be asleep, as it's already 10:00 p.m. I feel confident about this because I've dosed both boys with Dimetap, an antihistamine that should keep their ears from building up pressure at takeoff. The great side effect of Dimetap is drowsiness.

Well, my hopes don't work out. Kurt goes to sleep very quickly, but Kory has an idiosyncratic reaction to the Dimetap. Instead of getting sleepy, he's energized and stays wide-awake on this, his first flight. ALL the way. And he never lets up on the unfortunate man in the seat in front of him. For nearly six hours.

I offer to change places with Kory, but the man says, "Why would I want my wife or kid to put up with this? Just stay put, and don't speak to me again." He never stops looking back at me, rolling his eyes. I can't blame him. In later life, karma will catch up with me, and I will be the one sitting in front of the kicking child many times. For the entire trip, Kurt sleeps peacefully. At least Kory is quiet. He just can't sit still, and he never does sleep. So neither do I.

We finally arrive, and I lug the suitcases from baggage claim to the nearby train station. More than once I have to rely on the charity of shopkeepers to watch my children while I ferry my bags one at a time in a chain of moves. I am unable to find a porter to help me move the luggage from baggage claim to the train station.

Finally we're all on the train to Oxford. It's a short train ride and so scenic, with morning light filtering through clouds onto a fairy-tale scenery of castles, spires, pastoral fields, and cottages. We're met at the station by wonderful Melinda, whose little car groans with our family and bags. Kurt and I sit in the backseat with 140 pounds of luggage on our laps.

At Melinda's home we are graciously received and nurtured. She takes us to all the wonderful colleges of famed Oxford. I never had any idea of the brickwork, exquisite lacelike ornamentation, wood paneling, and gardens that make up Oxford University and the surrounding area. Our week with Melinda passes quickly, and she and I catch up with our lives. I'm saddened to hear of her child, recently born two weeks early, who died because of immature lungs. Within a very few years new techniques for dealing with these early births would be developed, and by 2010 even babies born as much as eighteen weeks early can be saved.

Everything about England is new to me. I've never been to Europe or Great Britain, and I will spend the summer immersing myself in the rich history of the place, both in fiction and nonfiction, as well as in our travels. My ancestry is all from England. My maiden name is Thatcher, and my mother's maiden name is Lyman. All my ancestors arrived in America between 1632 and the 1700s, so it's even more interesting for me to begin to understand my roots.

The time passes quickly, and before I know it, the day arrives for Karl to call. At the prearranged time, I am sitting in a comfortable rocker by the phone. No call. I sit there for the entire day so as not to miss his call. No call. I call home to speak to the house sitter. She says that Karl hasn't been home. He should've arrived there yesterday, but no Karl.

Finally I give up and accept he will not be calling today. I feel adrift. We're stuck with staying home and no sightseeing until he calls, but I can't find him and resolve things. Next day, same scene. No call. Not at home in Burnsville.

The next day, finally, at six in the evening, he does call. He offers no explanation for not calling or where he's been. "I just forgot. Honk, honk. But it's okay. I'm ready to come now," he says.

Well, at least we know he'll be in tomorrow, and we go down to London to meet him at the airport. I have the kids and all our luggage in a rental car. Finally his flight arrives.

At the gate, we see him coming up the ramp, carefree and cheerful. When he sees us, he won't meet my eyes, and he isn't especially warm with his hugs, even with his kids. I know this routine. It's called a guilty conscience, and I've seen it so many times before, it isn't even worth making a scene about. We're all together in England, and I decide to make the best of it. Our family is about to have an amazing vacation, and I don't want to waste time.

We spend the day at the famous London Zoo. The kids are excited and exclaim at each new discovery. Both Karl and I enjoy the whole day. After an overnight in a nearby bed-and-breakfast, we board the train to Cardiff. Our London exploration has been cut short by three days because of Karl's late arrival. For me it will be fine because the boys and I'll be back often to continue the sightseeing, but Karl has missed everything except the zoo.

On the train en route to Cardiff, Karl and I play cribbage and chat. The boys are thrilled with the train and love the pastoral scenery, so they are quiet. I begin to comment on things we saw yesterday at the zoo. Karl just looks puzzled.

"I really loved the aardvark. What a strange animal. What was your favorite animal yesterday?"

No response, just a blank look at me.

"Were you scared when Kory got up on the wall enclosure around the bears den?"

No response, just another blank look.

Finally, Karl says, "What the heck are you talking about?"

"Karl, don't you remember all the stuff at the zoo yesterday?"

"You must be crazy. We didn't go to a zoo yesterday."

I sit back and shut my mouth. My heart is racing. What's going on here? I'm really frightened. I realize I have to accept that Karl now has some brain problem, either from too many concussions or from alcoholic blackouts, which I now know much more about, or both. I'm stunned and saddened. I know from my training that he's never going to be the same, never going to be all there again. I'm really grieving for him and for all of us and don't attempt to have any conversation the rest of the trip while I try to digest this new disaster. I feel sick about it.

Later in life I will suffer a moderate concussion after being hit by a pickup truck that sped through a stop sign. The drunk driver—this would turn out to be his tenth DWI—broadsided my car right at the driver's window, knocking me unconscious. I was taken to the hospital via ambulance, and my totaled car was towed away. I have no memory of the x-rays, glass removal, or suturing up and down my left side. Although I appear to be conscious after ten minutes, because I converse and answer questions appropriately, it will be many hours later before I actually know where I am or what's going on around me. The time in-between is lost.

And yet I'll behave "normally" during this lost time. Everyone thinks I'm completely conscious. It'll be a good lesson for me in how there's an automatic behavior part of the brain that does not require the conscious knowledge of current events or circumstances. Normal behavior and responses are programmed in. After this accident, I have a clearer understanding of how Karl could continue to play challenging cribbage with me on the train trip to Wales, although something was clearly going haywire in his brain.

What I do know, once again, is that I cannot stay in this marriage. I can't tolerate all his self-destructive behavior and his infidelities, and I can't watch Karl deteriorate or, even worse, be killed or injured. Once again I resolve to bail out, and soon.

Even so, we have a pleasant nine days together before he must return to America and head to training camp. We play cribbage, make love, sightsee, eat, and make friends around the duplex in suburban Cardiff where we're situated. It's a good time for all of us, and I'm sorry when the day arrives to prepare for Karl's departure the next day.

On his last night, we're returning from the central shopping area in Cardiff when I ask, "Karl, the next-door neighbors would like an autographed picture. Could you give them one before you go to bed tonight?"

He looks blankly at me—he's driving—and out of nowhere he whacks my forehead at the hairline with his balled fist. I'm knocked speechless. He's never hit me before, and I don't know where this came from. We weren't fighting or even disagreeing about anything.

Blood streams down my face from the inch-long gash in my hair, caused by his wedding ring. He doesn't even react at first, and I tell him to turn the car around, because I have to go to the emergency room. I walk into the royal infirmary alone. Karl waits in the car. My tale to the emergency room doctor has something to do with a sharp cupboard door. They put in four stitches, give me a few pain pills, and send me on my way.

On the way home, Karl says, "I'm so sorry, Janny. I don't know what came over me. Can you forgive me?"

Forgiveness is easy, staying with him isn't. I remember what I saw at his house the first time I was there, and I've already learned something about the fledgling field of information about domestic violence. I know for sure I will never be a victim of this particular problem. One whack is all there will be for me.

In fact, Karl's behavior has helped me understand an essential for the rest of my life. I am not going to be a victim of anything. I've had to accept that bad things really do happen in life. My golden cocoon is over, and I will be thrown about by life's challenges, just like everyone else, but I'll refuse to be a victim. Karl has helped me to understand I can always make the choice to move forward, rather than create an identity for myself as "poor Jan." For this I will always be grateful to him, as I'd never pondered this idea before.

As I'm packing his clothes for the return home, a receipt falls from his pocket. It's a registration form for Mr. and Mrs. Kassulke at a Chicago airport hotel for the exact time when he should have been home in Burnsville and calling me.

I show it to him. He grabs it, crumples it and tosses it into the wastebasket. "It's just a mistake. I have no idea what it's about."

That's the extent of our conversation about his mysterious disappearance for two nights. I know better than to ask more. He'll only deny everything.

In the morning I give him clearly written instructions about when to pick us up at the airport when we get home. He will have been home from training camp for a week.

⌁

DURING THE summer, the boys and I have an absolutely delicious time. I go to school for three or four days a week, and we travel the rest of the time. Before our time is over, we'll have seen all the sights of Wales, including the magnificent Carnarvon Castle area and the beautiful *How Green Is My Valley* Brecon Beacons mountain range in south Wales. Everywhere we go we stay without prior reservations at wonderful bed-and-breakfast establishments. We're nomads, and it's great.

We tour Stonehenge (both boys climb on the monument) and Tintern Abbey (the boys climb on the walls). Kory steps into the middle of the changing of the guards at Buckingham Palace, and then wails in the basement of the Tower of London. He's terrified of the darkness with the prison cells and suffering mannequins. Both boys delight at a complete miniature town tourist attraction in someone's backyard. It's remarkably accurate, even to the replicated tiny town in the backyard of a miniature house.

We'll also explore southern England, right down to Brighton Beach and Bristol, and from London to the western coast, between Wales and England. We have so many adventures and so much fun, I don't think much about Karl's lack of communication. We get one letter from him; I send four, all with complete instructions on picking us up at the airport and also filled with news of what we're doing. I call him once when he gets home from training camp to confirm our arrival plans.

One night we arrive at Hampton Court Palace, and we stay in a nearby bed-and-breakfast over a bar. Both boys are asleep, and it's 2:00 a.m. when I head down the hall to the bathroom. I am sitting on the toilet when suddenly, from the small hole through which the sink pipes exit, a large rodent emerges. I'm alarmed. I have no experience with this kind of thing. I've seen mice before, but never anything as large as this rodent, and certainly not when I'm trapped with it in a small bathroom.

I stamp my feet, thinking it will scare the rodent off, but it just keeps coming toward me. I leap off the toilet, slam the door behind me, and race downstairs to the bar, still in my nightclothes. All the men lift their beer glasses to me when I run in. The lady owner is behind the bar.

"Quick, there's a large rodent in the bathroom. It scared me to death!"

"A rodent? What do you mean? Was it a rat?"

"I don't know. I've never seen a rat."

She thinks for a moment, then says, "Was it about eight inches long? Was it white with brown spots? Did it have any tail?"

I tell her she's perfectly described it.

"Oh, love, you've found Chauncey, our sweet little guinea pig. He's been missing for three months. Quick, let's go get him."

Sure enough, it is Chauncey, who seems very happy to be found. But I'm not able to sleep the rest of the night.

In the morning, the owner says, "Love, we're so glad to have Chauncey back. Here's your bill. I cut it in half."

The Welsh people prove hospitable beyond all expectations. I quickly learn not to admire anything in the house of Dr. Jones, my sponsor. He'll just hand it to me as a present. I'm acutely aware that I'm earning more working part time in a lab than he is as a doctor, and my salary when I start my internship will be nearly twice what he earns after thirty years of practice as a physician.

At the medical school, I pick up some examination and treatment tricks that will serve me well as a doctor. The doctors here do some things differently, and they are clever and cool ideas.

One day one of my molars cracks in half. It doesn't hurt, but I figure, "Why not get it fixed while I can get it done on the National Service?" I go up to the new dental school at the Heath (a suburb of Cardiff). It's a gleaming new building, not a historic one like the Royal College of Medicine in central Cardiff. When the dentist looks in my mouth, which includes one gold filling, he says, "I don't recommend we do the fixing for you if the tooth doesn't hurt. We could never hope to match the fine dentistry in your mouth. I'd get it done when I got home if I were you." I'm surprised at this. It's my first understanding that there are many levels of dentistry, and standard American dentistry is quite different than standard Welsh dentistry.

"But," the dentist continues, "since you're here, and since you're a medical student, do you mind if my students look at the dentistry in your mouth? You understand how important it is for them for teaching purposes?"

Of course I allow it, but I'm not prepared for the two hundred or so folks who stare in my mouth over the next several hours. My jaw aches when it's over, and I feel like a largemouth bass. Glad I could provide a thrill, though.

During my few days at school each week, the kids play with the neighborhood children. Though later in life both sons will complain that they remember little of this trip and wish they were older when we did it, they will retain some memories. Kurt, for instance, will for many years say "i'ther" instead of either and "ni'ther" instead of neither. Both boys will start their races with "ready, steady, go," instead of "get ready, get set, go."

Too quickly, my rotation is done at the medical school, and we move on for some more sightseeing. First, we go to Edinburgh for the famous Edinburgh International Festival, a celebration of all the arts. We attend several concerts and plays and tour the spectacular castle. The biggest memory for us all is a concert by the London Symphony. Our seats are on the stage behind the orchestra, and I get to watch the conductor, Andre Previn, close up, as if I'm in the orchestra. What a thrill.

Next, we head to Paris because we'll fly home from there. We find a bed-and-breakfast near the Luxembourg Gardens. Kory has a great time washing his feet in the bidet in our bathroom—something new. Amazingly, and quite by accident, we find another University of Minnesota couple at the breakfast table, where we're wolfing down hot chocolate and croissants. We see the sights of Paris and visit some friends—ever try to see the Louvre in three hours with two restless boys?—and I am attacked on the street and molested by a man who grabs my breasts, slams me up against a wall, rubs himself roughly against me, then runs off laughing.

At this time, we do not find many Parisians who are very friendly to Americans. Even charismatic and beautiful Kory cannot seem to melt their hearts. At one point on a boat tour on the Seine, Kory is standing on his seat to touch the underside of the many bridges we pass beneath. He is adorable and quite safe while he's doing this, but the Parisians scowl and frown at his behavior. So we're tired and very ready to get home.

We make it to our plane to Minneapolis. It's been a fantastic experience, but we're all glad to be getting back to our familiar life, and Kurt needs to get to school. He's already missed the first week of first grade.

We arrive in Minneapolis exhausted and get through customs. I look around for Karl, but he isn't there. I can't believe he would leave us in the lurch like this, so I call home.

He's there, stoned and smoking with my friend from medical school. He's completely forgotten today is our homecoming day. We must get a porter to help with our luggage, and then take a cab to get home.

And so this ninth summer of our marriage, our last together, ends on a very sour note.

Chapter 22

The Marriage Road Ends and So Does Medical School

S O KARL ENTERS HIS ninth season of pro football with the Minnesota Vikings in 1971. It's the usual season, with all the same suspects and characters. I will attend my last Vikings party. I'm avoiding most of them now, as the ones Karl chooses to attend are mostly drunken, drug-filled lost nights. But I do go with him one last time after a game. We're greeted at the door, and the host hands each of us a cigar-sized joint. We head for the basement, where the wives are chatting in a corner. I set the joint down and go over to be with the wives. The men have gathered and are doing something I've never seen before.

The guys are sitting around a large circular divan in the center of the room. They have a curious glass jar with an opening the width of the jar, perhaps six inches. In the bottom of this odd container are many, many ampoules, all the glass cracked open at an angle. I ask someone what this is. "It's amyl nitrite. They're called poppers," I'm told. I can't figure out why they're using this drug. It's used for heart patients for quick help in a heart attack, as it rapidly opens the arteries wide.

But then I watch. A guy sticks his head in the mouth of the open jar, inhales deeply, then falls back on the divan, seemingly unconscious. He stays immobile like this for about two minutes, and then sits up again. I ask what they're experiencing.

"Oh, man, it's ecstasy beyond description. It doesn't last very long, but it's very, very cool while it does. You should try it just before sex! You can't imagine what will happen then."

So the party is like that. Drugs abound. Booze abounds. Suddenly one of the Vikings officials descends the stairs into this basement mess. His face is stern. He confers with the host, then leaves, trying not to look at the scene of dissolution.

The host stops the party immediately, though it pretty well came to an abrupt halt anyway when management showed up. "Listen up, everyone. Management says the feds are looking for [name withheld]. Something about heroin and you and your roommate. Quick, get in the secret room."

With this the host pushes on a panel in the basement wall, and it amazingly rotates to reveal a completely secret room that none of us knew about. The player rushes in there, and the panel is closed. Just in time.

Eight federal agents crash into the basement, looking for the player. They also ignore the general scene of drugs (though there's been quite a lot of rapid toilet flushing just before they arrived). Their appearance is stereotypical: black suits, white shirts, black ties. There's not one glint of humor or good nature in any of their faces. They have a mission and are ruthlessly focused.

"No sir, I haven't seen him since the game. Why? Has he done something wrong?"

They don't find him and leave without a backward glance, like a pack of hounds on to a new scent.

This is enough for me. I don't want to be caught or arrested at this kind of party, or my career will be over before it starts. I'm shaken to the core at the disaster I could so easily have been dragged into. I can see the news now: "Medical student caught up in drug raid. Kicked out of school." So this is the last Vikings party for me.

This Vikings player becomes very addicted—to what selection of chemicals I never know for sure. What I do know is that as the years pass, he receives treatments for his addictions, and then speaks to kids to prevent their chemical dependencies. I read about his activities from time to time and am glad for him that he can use his challenges as lessons for others.

Sadly, many years later, in 2009 I run into him in downtown Minneapolis and greet him. He looks at me with that same blank look I saw in Karl toward the end of our marriage. I tell him who I am. He's cordial, but I can see he's not all there. His brain is fried, either by chemicals or concussions or both, but there's none of the vibrant personality I knew years earlier.

✤

I'M FINISHING my last senior electives in medical school. I just keep moving forward, knowing my marriage will soon end. I just don't know the means or the final reason. I've always trusted that the right time and opportunity will develop naturally for these kind of life changes. This is what I'm waiting for now.

On the surface, most everyone still thinks all is well. One journalist even does an article about us as a happy little family. The article ends up in print after we've separated. At this point, Karl and I don't fight or discuss our problems at all. He isn't always clear on events, anyway, and I just end up frustrated if we try. So we travel through our lives in superficial motion: making love, eating, smiling, playing with our children, speaking with journalists, and minding our separate careers. Neither of us bad-mouths the other. What would be the point?

After the football season, it's January, Vikings basketball season. At this time Karl is away for a week, playing in Montana. For many seasons now Karl's been gone for these events, often for a week or two at a time. He's become the manager and organizer as well as an enthusiastic player. I will later learn he also was making plans to buy a bar in Mankato. I don't know it at the time though.

At the same time, I've started a six-week elective rotation practicing as a student physician at a clinic in Shakopee, the same curriculum offering I helped set up in my early medical school days. There are several doctors there, but I'm assigned to Patrick J. Adams. This man is recently divorced, he tells me, and he's Burt Reynolds handsome, quite charismatic, twelve years older than me, and very quickly pursues me aggressively.

The affair begins innocently, with Pat taking me to Buck Hill in Burnsville to ski, as it's one of his passions. I've never been on skis, and Pat doesn't think it's necessary for me to have a lesson. So at the age of twenty-six, I trustingly strap on these long boards and stiff, heavy boots and take the short chairlift ride to the top. I don't know how to get off, though, so I promptly fall on my face. I can't believe anyone would expect me to get down this steep incline with these boards on my feet. I have no idea how to turn or stop. But down I go.

The sight of me careening down the hill dressed in my snowmobile suit, scared out of my mind and trying to keep my balance, seems to be very funny to Pat. Actually, it's cruel, as I'm petrified that I will be killed. I could have paid attention to this cruel streak, but I don't, thanks to my thoroughly acquired codependency. Pat himself would later coin a phrase I could use to describe myself here: "My head was up my ass."

But this is it, the thing I was waiting for. I fall, fast. I am so taken with his complete involvement with me, his cherishing me, his wanting me, all of me, right now. He's concerned, listening, gentle, funny, urgent, and aggressive in his total possession. It awakens so many deep feelings, so much I have missed for so long.

I start an affair with him. In the end it will turn out to be out of the frying pan and into the fire, but I'm not listening to reason. His lovemaking in his rented apartment is passionate, long, and skillful, and I finally experience an earth-shaking orgasm. Sex still hurts, but I've learned how to shift my body so the thrusts usually miss the painful areas. If one of those scarred, abscessed areas is punched, it stops everything dead as I curl up in agony for five minutes or so.

Just like that, we are together most of the day in our glowing little world. I'm home at night, of course. Very quickly, I've determined I'll leave Karl for Pat, as this is what Pat wants. He's persuasive, and I'm really not thinking very clearly, so caught up am I in the emotions of being wanted. Pat recognizes how vulnerable I am and swoops in for the kill.

He showers me with compliments, gifts, and endless attention. We eat at the best restaurants and make plans for exotic travel and fun. He's affectionate, a wonderful kisser, and never leaves me for a moment, except when I go home at night. And he's a kind and effective teacher and a very good doctor. I'm swept away with it all.

So, in one quick week, the long, sad dissolution of a marriage hits bottom, and it's decided. When Karl arrives home from Montana one night in January 1973, his suitcases are packed and sitting in the living room. I'm going to tell him to leave and will get a divorce.

I'm sitting up in bed when he comes into the bedroom. It's one o'clock. He stands in the corner. "What's going on, Janny?"

"Karl, I want a divorce. Your bags are packed for you. Please go."

He looks at his feet for a moment, then asks, "Well, can we have sex one more time?"

"No, Karl, we can't have sex ever again."

Again he quietly studies his feet, and then he looks at me. "You know, I've only been unfaithful with five women."

"I don't believe you, but it doesn't matter anymore."

Again a silence, and then he says, "You know, you were right about last summer. I picked up a woman, a teacher, on the plane from Iowa after the football camp. Instead of getting off the plane in Minneapolis, I went on to Chicago with her. We did stay in that motel. And you know what she said to me? She said my wife must be the luckiest woman in the world."

"Karl, listen to you. You're trying to tell me that when you were having an affair, your mistress said I am lucky, and you don't get the irony of that?"

"I guess I didn't think of it that way."

With that, he sighs, leaves the room, and walks out of my life. I think, "Not with a bang, but a whimper." Of course, once married, never truly divorced, for he will loom large in my life until the day he dies, and then some.

I've thought about the divorce terms for a long time. I have decided that Karl has sacrificed his body, his family, and his life for football, and I plan on at least giving him everything material he's earned from it: the house, a car, and all the furnishings, except my piano. I will not ask for alimony, just child support (fifty dollars for each boy per month), because the kids are going to stay with me.

We have a mutual friend, a lawyer, and ask him to represent both of us since we will not be fighting over anything. I ask to be allowed to stay in the house for the year I am interning, so as not to disturb the kids, and I'll pay the house payments during this time. All of these things are drawn up, and a judge makes it final in March 1973. We're divorced in two brief months.

One of the tough parts for me at the time is that some of the people around Karl are obviously pushing him into even more destructive, thoughtless behavior. I'm to see some of this when I go to the bank to add my monthly funds to each of the boys' college savings funds, a tradition I've insisted upon and with which Karl was fine. Both Karl's name and mine were on the accounts as custodians, but I'm absolutely gobsmacked to discover the accounts no longer exist. I insist on talking with the bank manager. I ask him how could this happen. He spreads his hands, staring at them. "Karl and some other guy came in and closed them. The other guy was telling Karl what to do."

The accounts have been drained. I know Karl would never think to do that; he cared about his boys too much. It's my first realization that Karl has fallen into dangerously greedy and wild hands very quickly, and once again my heart sickens with fear for his life.

Also, within two weeks after he leaves the house, he immediately purchases the previously forbidden Honda motorcycle, powerful and big. I'm even more afraid for him. Sometime after that, he's the owner of a bar in Mankato and will also become some sort of partner in a sports bar in Bloomington, The Left Guard. Many years later I will learn he also owned a bar in Mason City, Iowa. So all of his wild yearnings were achieved very quickly once the wet blanket of my disapproval was lifted.

And I, after two weeks of passionate lovemaking, find I am once again starting with fevers and severe pelvic pain. Pat examines me and informs me I have terrible abscesses and pelvic inflammatory disease. It seems the vigorous lovemaking has broken open some of the old, quiet abscesses from my previous gonorrhea, and I'm right back in trouble.

Once again I undergo two weeks of twice-daily penicillin shots and suffer incredibly. The pain never quits and is made much worse by any movement. It's as if someone has thrown tacks into my pelvis. The days of the orgasm are over until I finally have a complete hysterectomy and pelvic cleaning at age thirty-five. This surgery, which should take an hour, will require four hours of difficult separation of abscesses and scar tissue from the rest of my internal organs. The destruction from gonorrhea was extensive and shocking to the gynecologist. The bleeding is heavy, and I require transfusions. The gynecologist says, "I don't know how you've managed all these years with this much pathology. The pain must have been intense." That's an understatement. Until this surgery, I will suffer every time I have sex.

I still have some course work to finish, but I quickly discover that most of my Vikings friends are gone—just gone. This includes the players and their wives, plus most of the fans who have insinuated themselves into our life. This is not a surprise, but more of a sadness. It confirms for me the reality that I had become an extension of Karl's celebrity. Very few of the people in that life were my true friends.

This also extends to my church, the church where both boys were baptized, where I sang in the spectacular choir for years, and where the boys and I still attended on Sundays when we could. One day three men from Richfield Methodist Church show up at my door. I assume they are there to do a pastoral visit with me to see how I'm doing after the divorce and to encourage me.

Instead, they say, "Jan, we've been trying to reach Karl. Can you give us his phone number?" Not once do they ask how I am or do any pastoral visiting with me. It's as if I don't exist and never did exist in this church. I'm stunned, truly stunned. I know Pastor Chant would not ignore me in this way, but he isn't here.

The next day I call the church and transfer my membership to the little Methodist church in Shakopee. My parents have attended there when they visited town, and I will become a member there. There's a Sunday school for the boys, and as it turns out, they need an organist. Since I volunteer for this position and am not paid, I'm able to insist I will not accompany the choir, as that would require a Wednesday night commitment, which I cannot do. I will be on call at least every other day when I first go into practice, and I don't want to commit to any other time away from the boys. This arrangement works well, and I will be the Sunday organist at Calvary Methodist Church from 1973 until the church dissolves in June 2010.

The rest of the school year passes quickly. The boys don't seem to notice that Karl is gone. But soon he begins to miss his visitations, leaving the boys to sit on the curb and wait for him again and again, crying. He only arrives for about half of his scheduled visits, and he is always late. I'm angry about these slights to his kids. Many years later, when Kurt and Kory are in their forties, I ask them about those visits before Karl had his motorcycle accident.

They say, "Dad rode with us on his motorcycle just smashed drunk. He rode too fast, and we were scared. When we went to his apartment, he usually sent us downstairs to play pinball games in the game room while he was partying constantly upstairs."

I'm so upset when I hear this. The reality that the boys could have been hurt or killed hits me for the first time, and even these many years later I'm sad once again.

I must accept how very deeply into denial and codependence I was at the time. The thought that Karl would endanger the boys had never occurred to me. Of course I should have protected them more in this regard, and I feel so very fortunate they were unharmed. Not once did I ask them any of these details at the time, thinking to avoid any unpleasantness for them of having to tattle on their dad. I was already "the bitch" and never thought about getting child welfare to investigate. They could have been damaged in so many ways. I will have to live with that knowledge and be thankful every day that they survived.

⁘

Dᴜʀɪɴɢ ᴛʜᴇ year after our divorce, I hear all kinds of gossip, daily, from acquaintances from the Vikings days. Karl is engaged to a woman in Hawaii. Karl has broken the engagement. The woman has had an abortion. On and on, the rumors fly steadily, and people make sure I hear them all. Everyone at the medical school tells me stories. Later, my patients in Shakopee start their visit with "Did you hear about Karl?" People at church tell me stories. Everywhere I go, I hear of Karl's wild new life. Personally, I don't think it's a new life; it just isn't a secret anymore.

Karl isn't speaking to me much during this time. He's having a wild, good time without a wife to answer to, but I also know he's wounded by the divorce. I am too. And though I'm with a new man, and Karl's certainly with new women, I often feel as if we're still joined at the hip, and it isn't a good feeling. I will need a lot of healing in the future, and fortunately I will find a great therapist to help me with my sorrow and with my entrenched habits of denial and codependency.

Finally it's time for graduation from medical school. I've already passed part one of the national boards with scores in the high nineties percentile, so I can graduate, one of only thirteen women left in the class. The big day arrives. I've dressed in a long red dress with tiny white polka dots, red sandals, and a large, floppy red hat, my long hair flowing down my back. The medical school has made it optional this year to wear cap and gown, and I've opted not to in the usual antitradition spirit of the times. (Many years later, as president of the University of Minnesota Medical School Alumni Association, I will be at the podium once again. This time, I will address the graduating medical school class—and I will wear a cap and gown.)

I am surprised to not only get my diploma (which I still secretly wondered if I would receive, since I never completed calculus) but also to win some awards. First, I'm called back up onstage to receive the award for the most outstanding female student. This award has both a certificate and a check for five hundred dollars.

I'm truly honored, surprised, and delighted. Then I'm called back again a third time. This time it seems I've won the medical school research award. This one has a check for a thousand dollars! Wow! And the real irony here is that the person who wins second place is the man who called me a big horse when we were both in undergraduate microbiology. So without ever doing anything or planning any revenge on him, I have won, and he must take second place, which has no money award. What a day! I feel vindicated.

Graduating is almost anticlimactic for me, though. The past several months have been so full of turmoil, confusion, and disappointment in people, and I'm entering a new, unknown life with Pat, another book entirely. I only have one week off before I must start my internship at Minneapolis General Hospital. I'm sad, without a doubt, and wish my only emotion would be joy at fulfilling my dreams, but it's not to be.

My marriage failed, and I must live with that. And living with it means somehow being reminded every day by someone who wants to talk about Karl. This will happen all of my life, but it gradually gets less.

Ron Pitkin writes a book with Karl in 1981 that enjoys a great deal of popularity in Minnesota, and this stirs up a fresh round of people talking to me about him. When one is a celebrity or married to one, the entire world forgets about any boundaries and will ask or remind you of the most personal things. When the book is published, many will comment about what it says about our wedding day or other such events, and they especially will wonder if I've talked with Karl lately. And how is Karl? Do you see him often? Do the boys see their dad often? Did you see Karl's award ceremony on the television? I heard Karl is in the hospital. Did you hear Karl is speaking at the Burnsville school next week?

Many still, I can see, get a small thrill about talking with me about Karl, even though I am his ex. Even as late as 1997. In that year, a woman comes to my office for the first time. When I finish my examination, she says, "I read the book, you know." I'm not sure what book she's referring to. It's been awhile since anyone mentioned Karl. But sure enough, she's talking about Karl's book twenty-four years after our divorce.

Karl and I had been together during some of the most exciting years of his life. He made it in a tough sport, received honors, played fearlessly, and competed in a Super Bowl. He traveled to exotic places, was treated like royalty, and was recognized as a hero everywhere he went.

He had a storied life during our marriage. During that time, we both grew up but apart, as I knew we must. I finally could not live with the drinking and infidelities and sure knowledge he would get hurt or killed by his behavior. That he stayed in my heart as a good man at the core and the father of my children is a guarantee. As the years passed, I chose to remember that part of Karl.

~~~~~~~~~~~~~~~~~~~~~~~~~~~~~~

Chapter 23

Internship and the Accident

*J*THROW MYSELF INTO my internship year. I've already had many clinical rotations at Minneapolis General Hospital, and this is my dream hospital for an internship. It's the level-three hospital for Hennepin County. This means all the most serious cases from the suburban hospitals all around are brought here for advanced care. At the same time, all the indigent care also shows up here.

Of course there is the University of Minnesota hospital complex (which I did not choose because family practice still isn't a very honored specialty there) and Ramsey County Hospital (too far). I've had rotations at all these hospitals, and I'm so lucky to be at Minneapolis General. Later it will be a gleaming new megahospital and renamed Hennepin County General Hospital, but for now it's an out-of-date building where excellent medical care is dispensed under less-than ideal conditions.

I'm undertaking a rotating zero internship. This means I will spend equal time through all the rotations: surgery, obstetrics-gynecology, neurology, psychiatry, pediatrics, internal medicine, and emergency room. I am now responsible for my patients and make the decisions regarding their care, although everything I do will still be checked by a resident or staff physician.

This is still a brutal time to be an intern. The hours are unbelievably long. Common shifts are twelve to sixteen hours long, and the jangling phone often keeps me from more than a few moments of sleep. Interns are expected to deal with all problems first. If there is something that needs extra help to manage, then a resident may be called.

There is still an energy about the internship that's almost like a hazing. It's a trial of endurance and would not be possible were it not so interesting. (In truth, the hours are gentle compared to the hours and fatigue necessary to actually be one of the rare women in family practice.) Years later, research will demonstrate that this type of internship causes more medical mistakes and more disasters for the interns from lack of sleep and gross fatigue. The hazing years will end sometime after 2000, and internships and residencies will become much more humane.

But I am enjoying all the rotations and still learning every day. During this year, a new specialty will be developed—family practice—that supersedes the old general practice title. To be a family practitioner, however, requires an additional two years of residency after an internship. But for three years there will be a grandfathering stage, when all GPs can take the family practice board exams. If they pass, they will be specialty certified. As the years pass, insurance companies will not reimburse MDs who do not have specialty certificates, so certification is critical.

I am, quite frankly, very tired of school. I want to get on with my life, so I elect to do just the one-year internship, then take part two of the national boards, which I must pass in order to be licensed, and then take the family practice board exam, which I do pass. So I concentrate on my internship in order to be ready to jump into practice in Shakopee as soon as I graduate.

The year is filled with stories. This is the year when the idea originates of a completely equipped ambulance ready to handle an emergency when a patient is picked up. This means that lifesaving measures can be taken quickly, rather than waiting until the critically ill patient arrives at the hospital, with precious time and lives lost during transport, because nothing was done to help the patient until arrival. This is a radical new idea, one strongly developed at Minneapolis General. These early new ambulances are made from converted bread trucks, and they're very unbalanced and top-heavy due to all the medical equipment on board. They aren't created for high speeds, and they're staffed by interns; emergency medical technicians (EMTs) are a creation of the future.

One day during my emergency room rotation, I jump into the ambulance to ride all the way to Edina to pick up a forty-year-old man who has collapsed after a game of golf at the Edina Country Club. When we arrive, he isn't breathing and has no heartbeat. His buddies are standing around, scratching their heads (it will be a few years before everyone is encouraged to learn CPR, and even more years before all public places will have portable defibrillators at the ready). The fellow is ashen and has dilated and fixed pupils—never a good sign. We hear he's been collapsed beside his golf cart for about seven minutes. I begin CPR and intubate him, and the ambulance driver and I get him on the cart and into the ambulance. I'm frantically continuing CPR with chest compressions and ambu-bagging (forcibly breathing) as we hurtle down I-35W to Minneapolis General, sirens wailing and red lights flashing. CPR is hard work, especially since the man is obese, and my sweat is dripping onto his pale face.

Suddenly, fire erupts from beneath the front hood of the ambulance, and flames fly all the way to the back of the truck. The driver shouts to me through the opening into the medical work area, "What should we do? What if we explode?"

I have to make a split-second decision, and since we are totally gonzo at Minneapolis General, I shout, "Keep going. Call the ER and tell them about the fire." And I pray that we don't all die from my decision.

We are perhaps only four minutes from the hospital. The fire is getting larger and larger, and the driver is having some trouble seeing through the smoke and flames. My patient is just beginning to respond to CPR with a heartbeat. We can't stop here. If we do, he will die. I haven't even had time yet to put in an IV or administer any of the necessary drugs to stabilize him.

So we race to the ER, sirens screaming and completely aflame at the front end, and squeal into the ambulance courtyard on a two-wheel turn. What a surprise! The courtyard is completely filled with foam to put out the fire, which it does. When the ambulance hits it, it feels like driving into pillows. The emergency room orderlies run through foam up to their chests with a litter to get the patient into the hospital. He survives. I take a deep breath, glad we didn't all die in an explosion.

In the next year, an intern will be killed when one of these ambulances turns over on a fast corner. The vehicle design is improved after that.

&ty;

THE EMERGENCY room is certainly the most exciting rotation. This is where gunshot wounds, domestic abuse, auto trauma, and terrible tragedies of needless violence all come. It all requires quick thinking and rapid action and the ability to speak to the traumatized, recently bereaved, and scared-to-death people who populate such a place.

Sometime after I've finished this rotation, I receive a call to come down to the ER. A patient is asking for me and refusing care from any other doctor. I can't imagine what this is about, but I leave my internal medicine rounds and go down to the ER. There, waiting for me, is R, the same R who has been so in love with Karl.

He has been beaten, especially around the face. His expensive clothes are torn and filthy.

"What happened, R?"

"Will you fix me up? I don't want any other doctor."

"Okay, the emergency room will let me do the suturing. But what happened?"

It seems R had been in a bar, drinking hard. (It's just barely noon right now). Somehow he got into a fight and was beaten, robbed, and totally trashed by several men. So here he is.

It takes me much of the afternoon to repair all the tears and gashes in his previously handsome face and body. Fortunately, he doesn't seem to have any broken bones or internal injuries.

"How's Karl? I miss him so much. Do you think he still thinks about me?" R talks about Karl the entire time.

I will see him one final time a week later to remove all his stitches. He's bruised all over, with multicolored patches covering his face and body. After that, I will never see R again. His story does not end well.

Karl played with fire with R and refused to see how heartbroken R was. Karl just wouldn't listen to anyone about him. Most of R's friends blamed Karl when R started drinking again and lost his dignity and his business. I can't say R's downturn was entirely Karl's fault, but he sure didn't help things.

Finally someone tells me that R moved to another city with his wife. I will hear they started a new business there that was quite successful, but R's grief at his entire life became too much for him to handle, and he went into the garage, turned on the car, and killed himself.

After many challenges and delights, this interesting but tough year is over. I am certified and licensed as a doctor. Again, it feels anticlimactic. I'm sorry to say good-bye to my hospital family, knowing I'll very rarely see any of them again.

Immediately, I move with the children to a house in the country outside Shakopee, because I'll have one week off before I start work at the clinic there. Pat and I are building a house in the country, and we'll rent until it is completed. As soon as I move out of the Burnsville house in early June, Karl moves into it. He's not there for long, though, before the thing I have dreaded for so many years finally happens.

⁕〜⁕

IT'S JULY, and I am home with the kids in Shakopee when the phone rings.

"Jan, this is Bud Grant." I'm speechless. Why would Bud Grant call me?

"Karl has had an accident. Bring the kids and come immediately to the Methodist Hospital emergency room."

"Bud, what's happened?"

"Just come quickly," he responds.

I gather up the boys, and we drive without talking to the emergency room at Methodist Hospital. There we are quickly ushered into a room where Karl is lying on his back on an examining table in the center of the room. There are no doctors or nurses present, no IVs, no oxygen. Just Bud Grant, Karl, and us.

Bud has tears in his blue eyes. Karl is conscious, and I kiss his cheek several times. There is no blood; he's apparently been cleaned up.

"Oh, Janny, it's so good to see you. Bud, do you know my wife, Jan? And Kurt and Kory, you rascals! How's your summer going?"

He doesn't honk, he just smiles, and Bud Grant looks away. Just then I see the x-rays on the light box on the wall. They show a totally smashed spine. I look at Bud. "Are those Karl's x-rays?"

"Yes, they are."

I know what this means. Karl is paralyzed, at least from the waist down. This is the end of life as Karl knows it. "Bud, what happened?"

"Karl and a friend were on Karl's motorcycle. They had changed places, and the friend was driving. They hit a car at high speed, and Karl was thrown between fifty and a hundred feet."

There will be many rumors later that the driver, or both Karl and the driver, were impaired at the time of the accident. But I will never know if this is true.

Karl seems to be fading in and out of consciousness. I give him one last kiss on the cheek, and the boys squeeze his hand. Then it's clear there's nothing I can do, and Bud called us in so the boys could see Karl one last time in case he died. I hug Bud, who is not known as a demonstrative man, and we leave. A new chapter has begun. First, we will have to see if Karl survives. Then he will have to rebuild a life—a new one. I will not see Bud Grant again until Karl's funeral thirty-five years later.

The next week is hell for us all. The media is in a frenzy, and the rumors fly. Was the driver impaired? Were they both impaired? What really happened? Will Karl survive? (He's slipped into a coma now that lasts for months.) Why didn't his wife stay married to him and keep him stable? This surely wouldn't have happened if she'd kept him under control.

Fortunately, it's summer, and the boys don't know anyone in Sha-kopee, so they are protected from most of it. Of course, people do talk to them and ask questions.

It's touch and go. Everyone knows Karl is paralyzed, but no one knows if he will wake from his coma. Months pass, and we visit him from time to time, but he is not responsive. Finally, he wakes. For reha-bilitation and introduction to his new lifestyle, he's transferred to the University of Minnesota Hospital.

Odd things still happen, as they always will with Karl and me. For instance, one day Dr. Rosenberg calls me to talk about Karl's sperm. "Do you think the doctors should take a sample of Karl's sperm and freeze it? You know, with no nerve connection, his sperm production will be gone soon."

Why am I being asked this? I don't know. A courtesy, I guess. I tell Pearl, "I don't have any say regarding Karl's medical care. The folks there will have to decide this question." I will never know what they decided about this particular problem, and I don't want to know.

It's finally time to take the boys to see Karl, something we will do sev-eral times while he's at the university. When we walk into the room, where Karl has three roommates, all paralyzed, Karl breaks out in a huge smile. "Janny. Janny. Here you are. Guys, this is my beautiful wife, Jan. Isn't she great? And these are my two wonderful sons, Kurt and Kory."

I take his hand and kiss him on the cheek. I'm so glad to see Karl awake, but I'm mortally embarrassed he's still introducing me as his wife. Doesn't he remember we're divorced? We visit for an hour or so, an hour where my horror grows with each word out of Karl's mouth. I quickly see he is severely brain damaged and cannot remember what he has said fifteen seconds before. His humor is there, his laugh, his smile, but his words are like a broken record as he repeats himself over and over. The boys don't understand any of this. What's the matter with Dad? Why is he talking this way? Why doesn't he get out of bed and walk with us? I must have many gentle talks with them about their dad, who will never be the same person again.

Meanwhile, in between visits to Karl, I'm heavily into practicing medicine in Shakopee. I am on call every third day, and since I am a rare woman doctor, my practice is full to overflowing. It's very hard for me to keep up with it or get any sleep.

Finally, Karl has finished his rehab and moves back to the house in Burnsville for a short time. But it isn't a good house for a handicapped person. The boys don't see their dad during this stage, as there's no one to pick them up, and those around Karl have made it clear I am persona non grata. They evidently don't feel that it's important to manage visitation with his sons, and I don't even know Karl's phone number.

Even though the boys don't see their dad, they must both speak of him almost daily in school as curious and impressed folks want to talk about him. Kory is in kindergarten, and Kurt is in third grade, so it's all very confusing for them.

I begin to realize how very deeply Kurt is struggling when he writes a haiku one day for a school assignment. To preface this, I must say that I have taken up rock climbing and have taught the boys as well, so they are well versed in all the terminology and techniques. They love to go with me to the cliffs by Taylors Falls, where we spend wonderful days climbing together.

So Kurt writes: "Handhold in solidest rock. / Gone in a second."

When I read this, I am very concerned for Kurt. After all, I'm not the only one who has suffered through all this. The kids have their own issues as well. A few days later, we are driving over the Shakopee bridge over the Minnesota River. Almost as if he's speaking to himself, Kurt says, "This would be a good place to jump."

That does it. These little guys have been through a lot with a famous but missing and puzzling dad, a mom who is a doctor—their friends all argue that that isn't true, she's a nurse—a divorce, some less than perfect baby-sitters, a new man on the scene, and a move away from their home and base of friends and school.

So I call Dr. Hilmer Carlson, the psychologist I refer all my patients to. He's compassionate and caring, and most of my patients improve greatly from his wisdom and help. Now I want his help with Kurt. Kurt begins to see Hilmer every week for the next few years. Kory does as well, when he gets a bit older. Hilmer releases them both when he feels they are back on solid footing.

Rumors are still flying about Karl. Many folks who cross my path in many parts of my life still want me to hear all of these rumors, so they make sure to tell me. There's wild partying going on in Burnsville. Karl is learning to drive with hand controls in his van. Karl has a girlfriend who was his nurse. Karl is getting married. Karl is moving somewhere away from Burnsville and selling the house. The house sold for $160,000. The National Football League is going to grandfather Karl into the pension plan, so he will have a very good yearly income, in addition to his Social Security disability.

⚬

THE PART about the girlfriend being Karl's nurse proves correct, and Karl marries Susan. Now, with Karl remarried, I enter some more challenging years. First, I receive a call one day from the archbishop of St. Paul. This Catholic cleric has sent me a questionnaire a week earlier. It is filled with personal questions about my life with Karl. Were we incompatible? Did we have trouble with our sex life? I can't see how any of this is the Catholic Church's business, so I toss it in the garbage.

Now the archbishop is calling. I'm sitting at my desk at work. "Dr. Jan, can you fill out the form, please? Karl and Sue want to be able to take the sacraments, but they can't unless Karl's first marriage is annulled."

"Are you crazy?" I ask. "Why would I answer these personal questions? Karl is basically Lutheran, and we were married in the Methodist Church. How does the Catholic Church have any say about whether this marriage is annulled?"

"Well, it's very important to Karl and Sue."

"What about my kids? Does that make them bastards?"

"No, no, it's only a little paper. It doesn't mean anything."

"Well, if it doesn't mean anything, then why bother with it at all? By the way, how many people are granted annulments who request them?"

"Well, of course, we have to carefully consider each case."

"How many?"

"Actually, most of them."

"What does that mean in percentages?"

"Well, nearly 99 percent are granted."

"Why bother with the exercise, then? Why not just automatically grant everyone an annulment? I find this whole thing more than just a little cynical. No, I will not answer these ridiculous questions. Our life together is none of the Catholic Church's business, and you're going to give him an annulment anyway, aren't you?"

"Well, yes, we are. If you won't cooperate, we'll just call you a hostile wife, which is plenty of reason for annulment."

Sure enough, I get a letter several weeks later announcing that the Catholic Church has officially annulled my marriage to Karl. This is just beyond weird to me. But it's just the opening round to a few years of weirdness.

Chapter 24

The Weird Years and All the Rest

 $\mathcal{A}$ s Karl and Sue settle into their life together, child visitation begins again. It doesn't go very smoothly for some time. The kids are not comfortable around this new version of their dad. Kory, in particular, is distressed at Karl's constant repetition. And somewhere in there, Karl and Sue have left the Catholic Church, now that Karl has been successfully annulled from me, and started active participation in a charismatic and evangelical end-times church, the Jesus People, which meets in the old State Theater in downtown Minneapolis.

Kory is quite distraught by all the talk of the world ending and "the Rapture." Each time he returns from visiting his dad, he cries himself to sleep, certain that the world will end in the morning. I am not happy about this. Why would Karl choose to scare his little boy like this? This is totally unlike the Karl I have known.

Visitation is bumpy, and it's clear for now that I am very unpopular, to say the least, in Karl's house. For whatever reason—I am not in this discussion loop at all—I'm taken to court several times over the next years for custody battles. Each time there is some concession: more visitation, less child support (which is never paid, anyway). But Karl and

Sue want full custody of the boys. Finally, when the boys are nine and twelve, custody is permanently settled: the boys will stay with me. In order to settle this chain of battles, I have to hire a guardian ad litem, an attorney to speak to the judge about the boys' wishes. This attorney does not consult either Karl or me—just the boys. The boys want to stay with me, so that settles it.

Meanwhile, Karl becomes a father again. I'm not privy to how this comes about, but it does. Susan has a little boy, Christopher, so Karl now has three sons. It's just speculation on my part, but I believe having their own child to raise takes the pressure off me. Life for all of us eases into a more peaceful time. The boys see Karl from time to time, and the period of hostilities seems at an end.

I will have very little personal contact with Karl for several years, but the boys and the media keep me pretty well informed. There is a Karl Kassulke Day at one of the football games. And the book about Karl comes out, stirring up media attention again. Karl seems to have settled reasonably happily into his new life with his new family, and I am glad for him and for them all.

Karl takes the boys to football games or they play cribbage. In a talk with Kurt and Kory while I'm writing this book, I will once again learn disturbing things that endangered their lives and once again have to reflect on my own high level of denial. Kurt tells me that at the football games, the beer vendors comped Karl with endless glasses, so that he was quite drunk by the end of each game. Riding home in Karl's handicap-equipped van, Kurt would comment, "Dad, don't you think you're going too fast? You have an awfully heavy arm there. Could you slow down?"

Karl's response was always, "Relax. Everything's just fine.

Kory tells me that when he became an adult, he had his dad's love of alcohol and usually took a bottle with him to see his dad, and the two of them always drained it. I don't know why, but I'd always assumed Karl stopped drinking after his accident. When I tell Kory this, he says, "Oh, no. Once an alcoholic, always an alcoholic."

Both boys say they feel Karl slowed down on his drinking as he aged, but he would still drink anything that was placed in front of him.

I continue to get sketchy reports of Karl. He's doing some kind of work with Blue Cross Blue Shield and is volunteering with the March of Dimes and other charities. The few articles about him now speak to his humor, his laugh, and his altruism. No matter what, we still seem to be joined at the hip.

The years pass. Occasionally Karl will show up in his wheelchair at one of the boys' games or wrestling matches or school plays or graduations. They're always happy to see him there, although they never really expect it.

+〜+

Years later Kurt graduates from Stanford and moves to Los Angeles, where he is finishing his master's degree in film production at USC. He'll eventually win an Emmy for his work on the television show *Ally McBeal*. And he's getting married. In Los Angeles. Karl can't take a plane trip, so after the wedding there, I plan a big splash of a reception in Shakopee.

It's a fine summer day. My yard is festooned with white tents, a band is playing, and there is catered food to die for. The cake—Kurt's favorite, from Wuollet's Bakery (with real whipped cream)—is a vision. All of the Kassulke family attends, including Karl, Sue, Christopher, Karl's mom, and his sisters (sister Kathy would soon die of alcoholism in her forties). We're all so glad to see each other. It's just like old times, catching up. The reception is great, and I'm so glad Karl gets to experience some of the joy of Kurt's wedding.

Still later, Kory graduates from the University of Minnesota. After singing with the Dale Warland Singers and the Minnesota Opera, among other stints, he decides to move to Wilmington, North Carolina, to get some work in film. He and his bride, Pauline, choose to get married in our Shakopee backyard. Karl and Sue and Christopher and all Karl's relatives come, and once again it's good to see them all. The yard is filled with happy people, white tents and a band, and scrumptious food. It's a gorgeous autumn day, and a special blessing seems to come from the big orange basswood leaves that drift into the hands of the happy bride and groom.

Life goes on, each of us striving to create the best we can for those we love. But now the consequences of our entanglements with chemical dependency will play out. In my life I've made a shrine to denial, I'm so clueless at times. Karl's dad was an alcoholic, his sister died of it, he himself is an alcoholic, and eventually I will learn that my beloved Kory is near death from alcoholism. Under the worst of circumstances, I'll discover that Kory had been drinking hard liquor—tequila was his poison of choice—since high school. Yet I never knew this until I saw him drunk—just once—when he was a senior in college.

When Kory's son, Dominic, was a month old, I went to Wilmington to visit. What I saw worried me enormously. Kory was drinking all day long and appeared drunk much of the time. It seemed like mostly wine, but in fact there were huge amounts of tequila also. Pauline was breast-feeding and was very frustrated with Kory and flustered with her new role as mother. I sat them both down and talked long about the need, right then, especially with their new responsibilities of a baby, for getting help with the alcohol. I talked about hitting the bottom, all the trouble that was coming down the pike, all the platitudes and AA wisdom.

They were hearing none of it. Kory had no interest in stopping drinking, and Pauline argued against him stopping as well. She insisted he should be able to drink wine at night. It would be several years before I learned she, too, was an alcoholic, though she did not drink during her pregnancy or while she was breast-feeding.

So I stuck my head in the sand for as long as I could, since there was really nothing I could do. The next time I went to Wilmington, it was because of a cry for help from Pauline: Kory was drinking to oblivion, over a gallon of tequila a day. I flew down and found all in complete disarray. My loving, gentle, kind Kory was a falling down, unpredictable, sarcastic drunk who had, with the help of his wife, ruined his business and their finances. He was bloated, red-faced, and with a liver so huge I could see it through his shirt. He was often picked up, dead drunk and filthy, for sleeping on the Atlantic beaches. His health was in critical condition, with high blood pressure, gout, and sky-high cholesterol.

Things were so unpredictable in their house, I never knew what would happen next. I tried to clean up the messes—cat urine was everywhere, dishes were piled high in the sink, and basket upon basket of unwashed clothes were piled on top of each other. I pleaded with Kory, talked about intervention with Pauline, and cried all night by myself. But I got nowhere. In the evenings, things were even worse, with Pauline also becoming hostile, screaming, and completely unpredictable. She was an alcoholic, but she had a different ritual from Kory's. Her drinking usually began in the late afternoon as she sipped from little bottles she carried in her purse.

I finally left a day earlier than I had planned due to the complete uproar that I was completely helpless against. I feared the worst, and every phone call became a nightmare.

A few days later, Kory slit his throat. Having failed by an eighth of an inch to hit an artery or major vein, he changed his mind and went to the emergency room for suturing. For a long time, he lied about it, saying he was drunk and fell on a stump, but he finally did tell the truth. By this time I was numb, sure I would lose my beautiful son and feeling helpless to stop it.

Then a saving grace happened, though it seemed like a disaster at the time. Pauline was behaving erratically at Walmart one afternoon, and they called the police. When the police arrived, she was in the car with Dominic, and they stopped her. She blew well over the legal limit, and they called Kory, who at that time had managed to get his drinking down to just at night. He'd downed two glasses of wine when the police called him to come pick up his son; his wife was headed to jail for DUI and reckless endangerment of her child. Kory climbed in the car and came at once.

They made him blow as well, and he tested just below the limit: .08. They were both arrested for DUI, and their child custody was suspended for the time being. Pauline eventually entered an outpatient treatment program and stopped drinking. Kory needed inpatient care for a month. It was a very long time before they had unmonitored custody of their darling boy again. Now Kory stays sober with very loyal attendance at AA, and I recognize my son once again as he emerges from the black haze of alcohol. It will still be some time before they dig out of all the financial trouble they created during their drinking days. I'm just truly grateful everybody survived.

The real saving grace in this whole mess is that the state of North Carolina stepped in and enforced treatment for both Kory and Pauline. In addition, they supported them in every way they needed until they got on their feet again. This is the huge difference between Karl's time and Kory's. The public is now openly aware of alcoholism and knows what to do to get help. Tolerance for drinking to excess has changed. It is no longer viewed as a minor issue, but a major one, one that ruins lives. Research now shows that alcoholism and its fallout wreaks havoc in every sphere and is a major health problem that needs vigorous treatment. Karl and I had no such information or help during our years together.

⌁

So many questions loom large now as I'm into my senior years. For instance, would I recommend anyone get married at age eighteen? No. Any individual at eighteen is still forming and will likely be someone completely different when they are thirty.

Would I have avoided early marriage if anyone had tried to stop me? No.

Would I recommend marriage to an untreated alcoholic? No.

Would I have tried to force Karl to get treatment if I knew anything about it? Yes.

Did I think I could get Karl to stop drinking because he loved me? Yes.

Would I have married Karl even if someone had told me he had a problem with alcohol? Yes.

Would I recommend anyone marry a celebrity, politician, or sports figure? No. This one requires some explanation. People in these arenas may start out as fine and true folks, but constant, often false, attention changes them, not necessarily in a good way, and their world becomes unreal. Rules that apply to others don't seem to apply to them. Can they resist all this? A few can, but most cannot.

My friend Gary was talking with me about this one night. He himself had wanted to play pro ball, but it didn't work out. As we compared Tiger Woods's recent problems to Karl's, he said, "Imagine you're Tiger Woods. You have a beautiful wife and two gorgeous kids. You live in a mansion and have a fortune. The public reveres and adores you, both for your skill and also for your apparent code of ethics. You have a giant picture window in your living room that overlooks scenery of unparalleled beauty. And every morning when you get up, five hundred vaginas are plastered against that window."

Such an allegory is not far off the truth, and very few can resist that constant siren call.

On that same subject, I was talking about Karl with Ron Pitkin, Karl's coauthor of the 1981 autobiography. Ron told me that Karl once said, in an unguarded moment, "I had a tendency to fall in love every weekend." Also, because the book had a focus on Christian redemption and would largely be sold by Christian bookstores, Ron told me he left out quite a lot of spicy material.

I don't know how many marriages can survive this kind of daily pressure cooker. Mine couldn't. Maybe I was too young. Certainly I was too naive. And definitely I was too haughty in thinking I knew everything.

Would I recommend an affair as an antidote to the pain and challenges of marriage? Definitely not! It might make for hot reading in a romantic novel, but in real life it is likely to add more pain to life.

Would I recommend jumping directly into another life relationship after a difficult marriage? Definitely not. Years are needed to process the lessons from a failed marriage in order to avoid repeating them.

These are some of the things I learned from my marriage to Karl, and I'm grateful for the lessons, for the fun and intimate times we were blessed with, and for our two great sons. Am I sorry I married Karl? Definitely not.

So as the years passed, the boys kept in touch with Karl by themselves, and I had very little contact with him anymore. Then, just in the middle of all Kory's troubles and Kurt's as well (though not with chemicals but money), I was diagnosed with cancer. I had not been feeling well for a year, and my training as a doctor told me I had cancer. I had all the symptoms of paraneoplastic syndrome, but the cancer was nowhere to be found.

Paraneoplastic syndrome is a set of maladies other than cancer that indicate a malignancy is probably present somewhere. I had a fever every day for a year, a low white count, and frequent illnesses like influenza A and B, which nearly killed me. In all the years I'd cared for folks with influenza, I'd never had a flu shot or become ill with the flu. Then I had multiple pulmonary emboli (blood clots in my lungs). Next was shingles—unbelievable pain. Finally, the cancer that could not be found turned out to be a rarity called a plasmacytoma, growing above the roof of my mouth. When it got big enough, it actually hung down the back of my throat, and the doctors could finally locate it.

The treatment was a draconian course of daily radiation. Though the radiation doctor spent over an hour preparing me for what to expect, I could not begin to imagine the tortures I was heading into. As usual, I felt very cocky after the first radiation treatment. After all, I hadn't felt a thing. Then, in the car on the way home, a hot headache started. By the time I got home, it felt like my brains were boiling inside my skull.

Eventually, I would have most every complication that could arise, pain beyond description, nine hospitalizations, endless transfusions, and a one-hundred-pound weight loss. And still the cancer didn't completely go away. I had to have an additional surgery to remove it, which also required removing some of the structures of the back of my throat. So now I can amaze folks by drinking water and bending over to have it run out my nose.

In September 2008, Kurt and his family arrive for a visit from Los Angeles. I am down so far that it looks like I may not survive. I'm shriveled into a bent-over ghost, like I've been in a concentration camp and cannot stand or sit for long. Sue calls and very graciously sets up a lunch with Kurt and his family. They haven't seen Karl for several years, either.

And the rest is history. For Karl, the cycle of life is complete. He has lived, loved, experienced joy with his three sons, become famous and infamous, raised hell, and in the end, found fulfillment with his family and his new, born-again Christianity. In a final irony, he outlived the average pro football player by twelve years.

For me, I will always carry the joys and scars of that amazing time so many years ago. I will always be grateful to Karl for the many lessons I learned while I was with him, for the exotic life and love we shared, and for our wonderful sons. And I will continue my own life for as long as I can, knowing that, if there is a heaven, Karl is there, playing cribbage and laughing.

Glossary

Alcoholics Anonymous, Adult Children of Alcoholics, Alanon, Alateen: twelve-step recovery programs, available worldwide, for alcoholics and their family members. Education regarding codependency and other associated behaviors is an integral part of these programs.

alcoholism: any condition that results in the continued consumption of alcoholic beverages despite health problems and negative social consequences.

chemical dependency: physical and psychological dependency on an addictive substances, such as alcohol or drugs.

chronic traumatic encephalopathy (CTE): a progressive degenerative brain disease found in individuals who have been subjected to multiple concussions and other forms of head injury, commonly from football, boxing, hockey, etc. Symptoms may develop around the time of the injuries or years later. Head trauma prevention is the only treatment. Symptoms include: deterioration in attention and concentration; memory loss; disorientation, confusion and depression; dizziness and headaches; lack of insight; poor judgment, aggression, and impulsiveness; overt dementia; slowed muscular movements and staggered gait; impeded speech and deafness; tremors and vertigo; death.

codependency: as it relates to chemical dependency, this is a tendency to behave in overly passive or excessively caretaking ways that negatively impact one's relationships and quality of life while enabling or allowing the chemically dependent loved one to avoid the negative consequences of their behavior. In this way, codependency prolongs the loved one's addiction.

cult of celebrity: the widespread interest in famous individuals that is manifested by a desire to follow a celebrity's life in every aspect, through various media attentions, or through concerted efforts to actually touch or enter a celebrity's life.

denial: one of the hallmark characteristics of codependency, denial is a defense mechanism used so that family and friends refuse to recognize or admit the behaviors in their loved ones that are already or are likely to cause serious work, school, relationship, family, or financial problems.

groupies: Most commonly associated with rock stars but present in the lives of all celebrities, athletes, politicians, etc. These individuals work tirelessly, creatively, and aggressively to get close to celebrities for sexual purposes or to fulfill a hope that the celebrity will find them fascinating and admit them into his or her life.